W9-AYH-693

WholeBody **Reboot**

WholeBody
Reboot

The Peruvian Superfoods Diet to Detoxify, Energize, and Supercharge Fat Loss

Manuel Villacorta, M.S., R.D.
with Sarah Koszyk, M.A., R.D.

Health Communications, Inc.
Deerfield Beach, Florida

www.hcibooks.com

Cataloging-in-Publication Data is available through the Library of Congress

ISBN-13: 978-0-7573-1821-4 (paperback)
ISBN-10: 0-7573-1821-5 (paperback)
ISBN-13: 978-0-7573-1822-1 (ePub)
ISBN-10: 0-7573-1822-3 (ePub)

Publisher: Health Communications, Inc.
    3201 S.W. 15th Street
    Deerfield Beach, FL 33442–8190

Cover photo © Joe Mazza Photography
Cover design by Larissa Hise Henoch
Interior design and formatting by Lawna Patterson Oldfield

CONTENTS

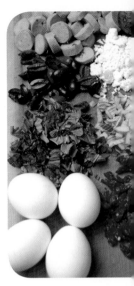

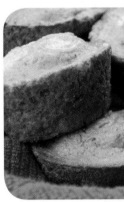

CHAPTER 4 Recipes

Breakfast

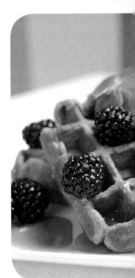

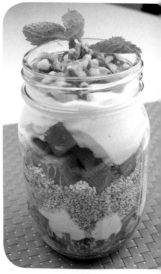

Main Dishes

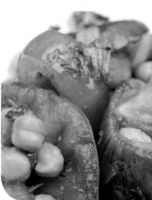

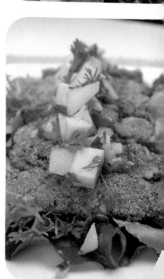

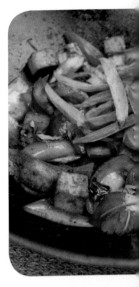

Shakes, Smoothies & Elixirs

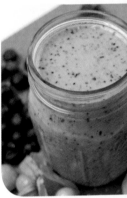

Salads, Sandwiches & Wraps

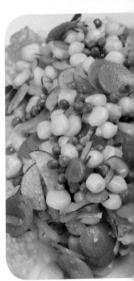

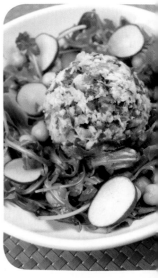

Soups, Stews & Curries

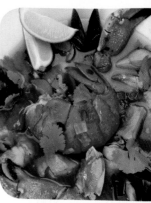

Snacks & Sides

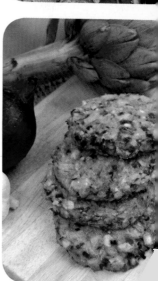

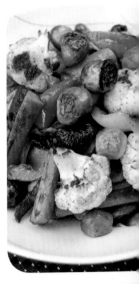

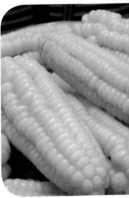

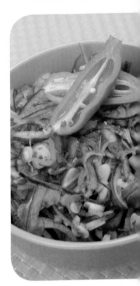

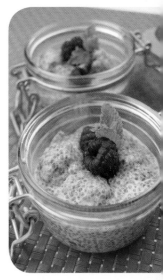

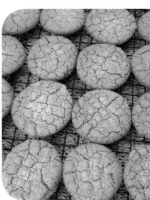

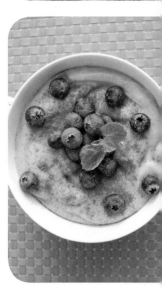

ACKNOWLEDGMENTS

The author wishes to thank the following people, without whom I couldn't have completed this project: Allison Janse, my editor at HCI Books, for believing in the project and pushing me out of my comfort zone and deeply inspiring me; Kim Weiss, for helping with PR and media strategy; Larissa Henoch, for working so closely with me on layout and design; and literary agent Andrea Hurst, for shepherding the project.

I would also like to thank my office team, whose dedication and support allowed me to focus on the project: Chenoa Bol, who spent many hours in the kitchen with creation of recipes and motivating food photography. I am grateful for Christy Greenwald for her outstanding energy and effort with the recipe nutrient analyses and assisting with meal plan development. Without your work, I couldn't have done mine.

I am eternally grateful for my dear friend and colleague, dietitian Sarah Koszyk, who accepted to contribute to this project. Her love for food, her involvement in the recipe creations, and her creative writing helped this book come alive.

Thank you to Jamie Farnsworth, foodie blogger from Girl Eats Greens, for her delicious recipes contribution.

I am always grateful to my family for your continued support and believing in my dreams. Finally, my deepest thanks to Papito for being my guinea pig with all my recipe development and trying all the food and smoothies. You are forever in my heart.

INTRODUCTION

A s a registered dietitian for more than sixteen years, I've heard—and helped people overcome—a myriad of challenges when trying to eat healthy and lose weight:

"I'd be thin if I went to bed at seven; it's the night bingeing that kills me."

"It's like after I hit forty, the pounds would not come off no matter what I did."

"I eat really 'good' during the day, but I'm hungry by dinnertime, and then it's all over."

"No matter what I do, I have this spare tire around my middle, and I'm sick of it."

With a specialty in weight management, I've seen yo-yo dieters, crash dieters, and countless numbers of diet fads and trends. I even had my own brief experience of struggling with college weight gain when I moved to the United States to pursue my studies at the University of California, Berkeley.

When I moved to the United States from Lima, Peru, I was far away from my family and clueless about how to cook and what to eat. Living with American roommates, I was introduced to grabbing a handful of cereal for breakfast while running out the door. For lunch and dinner, we scarfed down cold sandwiches or take-out. Sadly, not only was I gaining weight and lacking energy, I was missing my comfort foods from home. While it was apparent that this new lifestyle was not good for my health or wellness, I didn't know what to do about it.

Growing up in Peru, we always enjoyed homemade meals made with whole foods, which, unbeknownst to me at the time, incorporated powerful superfoods. This new way of living made me completely homesick, fat, and unsatisfied. Something was missing in my life, and that's when I said, "Enough is enough." I needed to reboot. I called my mom and asked her to mail me my favorite recipes (this was before e-mail). As soon as the mail arrived, I would rip open the letter, rush to the grocery store, and teach myself how to prepare my native dishes. Slowly, I began to get back to my normal weight. I felt invigorated, empowered, and revitalized. Back in the day, these Peruvian superfoods were very hard to find, but now they are readily available in the United States.

After realizing the strength that my native foods and diet gave to me, I did some research and discovered the reason why: the foods that I ate growing up are some of the cleanest, most immune-boosting, and most detoxifying foods on the planet.

Upon graduating with a degree in nutrition, I took my discovery a step further by devising an eating plan that incorporated twenty-one key Peruvian superfoods. Using a science-based approach, I introduced the plan to many of my clients, who experienced weight loss, improved moods, increased energy, and glowing skin. Peruvian superfoods were helping people feel on top of the world while cleaning up their systems from processed and packaged foods and toxins. Not only were they feeling amazing, my clients were losing weight and keeping it off. After just a short time, clients were expressing their successes:

"I wasn't able to lose weight before. But after doing your plan, I lost six pounds in a week and don't feel bloated anymore."

"Forget just the weight loss; my energy and sexual drive went through the roof!"

"My sugar cravings vanished. I lost ten pounds in eight weeks so I had to resize my wedding dress. This was beyond my expectations!"

This wasn't just a diet; this was a lifestyle change for people to recharge and reboot their entire system.

Now I am honored and excited to introduce the Whole Body Reboot plan and to educate you on how to maximize your weight loss and improve your health by enjoying exquisite recipes using superfoods. My clients' success has been my passion and my inspiration, and it continues to be so.

This diet is not a gimmick or a new diet trend. This is a way of living adopted from a culture that has thrived for centuries. Focusing on superfoods found in the Andes to the Amazon, my goal is to show you how to optimize your health and reboot your well-being from head to toe.

The *Whole Body Reboot* offers menus and recipes for everyone, whether you are vegetarian or vegan, you eat gluten-free, or you have no food restrictions. In order to provide such a comprehensive plan, I collaborated with my colleague and associate dietitian Sarah Koszyk, whom I've known for more than ten years and who has worked closely with me at my private practice. Sarah has also helped hundreds of people reach their health and weight goals, and we've been a strong team for a long time. In addition, she traveled to Peru with me to research this book; she stayed in my mom's home and experienced Peruvian culture firsthand with the locals.

If you are not currently accustomed to Peruvian cuisine, have no fear. We've incorporated many familiar American dishes into the meal plans, so you can comfortably cook simple recipes while expanding your culinary horizon with traditional Peruvian classics. We've also taken some not-so-healthy favorite American dishes and powered them up with a Peruvian superfoods makeover. Instead of using a prepackaged waffle mix, we've provided you with a quick and easy homemade recipe using sweet potatoes, a staple food in Peru. Everyone loves a good takeout pizza, right? Now you can make a homemade pizza from scratch using quinoa. Eating can be fun. Eating can be exciting. Eating can be a love relationship with your taste buds. Just like I taught myself how to cook, I'm going to teach you how to enjoy delicious, nutritious food with easy recipes so you can become a master chef in your own kitchen while losing weight and feeling great.

We look forward to sharing our wisdom and culinary skills with you in *Whole Body Reboot*. This plan is a delicious way to lose weight that will last for a lifetime. Expect to reboot your body, mind, and soul and to have more energy than you've felt in years. Get ready to experience a lifelong journey of amazing Peruvian superfoods that will keep you strong, healthy, and rejuvenated.

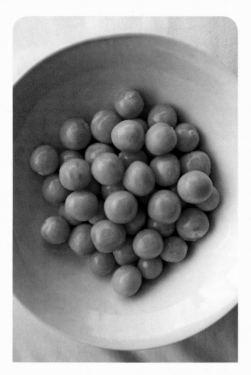

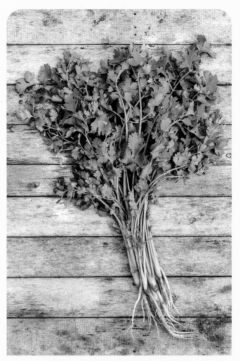

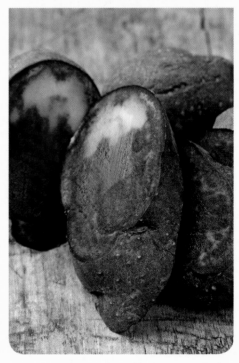

CHAPTER 1

WholeBody **Reboot**:
The Peruvian Superfoods Diet Plan

The key to the Whole Body Reboot diet are 21 superfoods. Superfoods are hardworking, functional foods that far surpass basic nutritional content. They are, quite simply, the cleanest, most powerful, antioxidant-rich, antiaging foods available anywhere.

Health Benefits of the Peruvian Superfoods Diet

Over the past few years, people have become aware of the health benefits of a Mediterranean diet, which focuses on eating fresh and whole plant-based foods; less meat; more fish; and heart-healthy omega-3s and monounsaturated fats. The many benefits of this type of diet include disease prevention, including cardiovascular disease, cancer, and diabetes; weight control; blood sugar regulation; and a reduced amount of inflammation. Our Peruvian-based diet is similar to the Mediterranean diet, but it will expand your options of flavors and tastes with a South American flare, bringing you a range of phytonutrients for optimal health. Unfortunately, not all Mediterranean food is nutritious in high quantities. Pizza, pasta, white bread, and endless bottles of wine can ramp up the calories quickly. That said, some Peruvian foods can also land you on the heavier side if consumed in large portions. However, by implementing the healthiest components of the Peruvian diet, you will lose weight while eating delicious food.

In the introduction, I shared about growing up in Lima and how I never opened a box of processed cereal for breakfast. Everything I ate was made from scratch using whole foods and a plethora of vegetables and fruits, whole grains, seeds, and naturally raised pro- teins. The true origins of the Peruvian diet are real foods and whole foods. Unfortunately, times have changed. Given the globalization of fast food and processed, packaged foods, the food climate has changed in Peru, especially in the cities. In supermarkets across the country, you now find processed foods and snacks, such as sugary cereal and cake mixes, jarred sauces, and packaged beverages, all of which contain preservatives and chemicals.

Peru, especially in urban environments such as big cities like Lima, has recently had an increase in the number of people who are overweight and obese. While doing research a few years ago, when I originally tried to find obesity and overweight statistics for Peru, I wasn't able to find anything before 1996. I even talked to members of the National Health Institute of Lima to help me find statistics. I was told that before 1996, no statistics were available because there was no obesity problem. The only statistics available before 1996 were for malnourished children in the Andes because of poverty. What had occurred in Peru in 1996 that resulted in the first statistics on overweight and obesity? The opening of the first fast-food chain! In addition, more supermarkets opened in Peru, which caused an increased consumption of packaged and processed foods. The introduction of fast and convenient food increased the weight of the population and changed the lifestyle of Peruvians. In the Amazon, the Andes, and less urban areas, whole foods and less processed and packaged foods are still used, but, unfortunately, life in the cities has changed.

According to a study done by Dr. Jaime Pajuelo of the Univer- sidad Nacional Mayor of San Marcos, the prevalence of metabolic syndrome in Peru is still lower, at 16.8 percent of the population having metabolic syndrome, when compared to 34 percent of the United States population. Metabolic syndrome is defined as a combination of medical disorders, such as a large waistline, high blood pressure, high fasting blood sugar, high triglyceride levels, and low HDL cholesterol, which can increase the risk of cardio-vascular disease and diabetes. The highest percentage of people with metabolic syndrome in Peru is located in the capital, Lima, at 20.7 percent. According to this study, this occurrence is most likely due to the influence of convenient and fast food over the past twenty years. Rural areas in the Andes still have a low percentage of metabolic syndrome (11.1 percent of the population), most likely due to less availability of convenient and fast foods. Nevertheless, as a whole, Peru still has 17.2 percent less people with metabolic syndrome than the United States, where fast and convenient foods were introduced at an earlier date.

According to another study by Dr. Pajuelo published by the Internal Society of Peruvian Medicine, the coast of Peru has a higher percentage of diabetes (2.9 percent of the population) than the mountains of Peru (0.9 percent of the population), likely because the coast contains more urban-populated areas, whereas the Andes are home to more rurally populated areas. The prevalence of diabetes has increased in the cities, most likely due to the increase of fast and convenient foods, bigger portions, and from dining out more often. This change in food choices may also be the reason why 10 percent of the US population has diabetes, whereas only 6.2 percent of the Peruvian population has diabetes, since people in the United States tend to dine out more often and use convenient, and fast foods on a more regular basis.

Sadly, the United States surpasses Peru's rate of obesity by 21.5 percent. In Peru, 14.2 percent of the population is obese whereas in the United States, 35.7 percent of the population is obese. Also, Peru has a greater difference of normal weight people versus obese people by nearly 33 percent in favor of normal weight people. In Peru, 47 percent of the people are normal weight with a BMI of 18.5–24.9. The United States has 31.3 percent of the population classified as normal weight. On the opposite trend, Americans have 4.4 percent more obese people than normal weight people—a negative number we don't want to see due to harmful health implications. According to research by Dr. Jaime Pajuelo in accordance with the Universidad Nacional Mayor of San Marcos and the National Institute of Health in Peru, the wide use of whole foods still has a positive effect on lower obesity rates in Peru when compared to countries that use more convenient and processed foods. Also, even though some food options have changed in Peru due to globalization and the introduction of fast and convenient foods in the major cities, history still remains strong within the culture, cuisine, and lifestyle of rural Peruvians who eat whole foods to reduce weight, lower risk of diabetes, and increase the rate of disease prevention.

Superfoods are still widely consumed throughout the country, especially in the Andes and the Amazon, where there is a lower incidence of metabolic syndrome, hypertension, diabetes, and obesity.

The 21 Superfoods

1. Ají
2. Artichokes
3. Avocado
4. Beans
5. Cacao
6. Camu
7. Chia Seeds
8. Cilantro
9. Kañiwa
10. Kiwicha
11. Lucuma
12. Maca
13. Papaya
14. Pichuberries
15. Purple Corn
16. Purple Potatoes
17. Quinoa
18. Sacha Inchi Seeds and Oil
19. Sweet Potatoes
20. Yacon
21. Yuca

Starting in the Amazon, you will find memory-boosting foods that improve brain health, such as sacha inchi seeds, which are high in complete protein and omega-3s. In addition, lucuma is a fruit rich in antioxidants and a good source of beta-carotene and calcium. Looking for an antiaging fix? Camu camu is extremely high in vitamin C. Moving into the Andes, you will find quinoa, kiwicha, and kañiwa, three seeds that are full of antioxidants, high in protein, and high in fiber. Pichuberries, found in the Andes, can provide you with 39 percent of your required daily vitamin D. Heart-healthy fats come from sacha inchi seeds, avocados, chia seeds, and flaxseeds. In addition, there are many immune-boosting spices in the Peruvian diet such as turmeric, an anti-inflammatory, cancer-preventing spice; ají, a spice derived from a pepper rich in vitamins A, B, and C; and capsaicin, which can assist with weight management. With all of these benefits, Peruvian superfoods truly offer an impeccable life of ideal health to reboot your entire body. Here are some of the general advantages that Peruvian superfoods can provide for you:

- Improved heart health by providing protection against hypertension, heart attacks, stroke, and high cholesterol. *Omega-3s* and *anti-inflammatory fats* can lower triglycerides and blood pressure and *monounsaturated fats* help reduce cholesterol and risk of heart disease

  Sources for omega-3s: sacha inchi seeds, flaxseeds, and chia seeds; a good source of monounsaturated fats: avocados.

- Disease-fighting *antioxidants* and *phytochemicals* act as free radical scavengers and contain anti-inflammatory properties that help reduce the risk of metabolic syndrome, cancer, diabetes, obesity, arthritis, and increase immune system support

  Sources: ají, pichuberries, purple potatoes, and corn.

- Antiaging **vitamins** and **nutrients** help increase vitality, longevity, energy, and improve memory, vision, skin, and sexual drive

  Sources: maca, lucuma, and sweet potatoes.

- Digestive health through **probiotics** and **fiber**, which help reduce bloating, gas, and stomach pain and cramps

  Sources: papaya, beans, and yacon.

Throughout the book, we will continue to highlight the benefits of these many foods. To better highlight them, here is a look at the whole-body benefits of these key superfoods:

In addition to the 21 Peruvian superfoods, we've also used some of the most powerful spices on the planet in our recipes, such as cumin, turmeric, curry, paprika, and cinnamon. Not only do these spices provide a wealth of health benefits, they are calorie free!

Benefits of Spices

Cinnamon: Seasoning a high-carb food with cinnamon can help prevent a spike in your blood sugar levels. Cinnamon slows the rate of gastric emptying after meals, steadying the rise in blood sugar levels after eating. Smelling the scent of cinnamon boosts brain activity by stirring our appetite cues, refreshing and warming the senses, and may even produce feelings of joy.

Curry: Growing evidence suggests that curcumin, the biologically active constituent of a main spice found in curry, may help prevent and treat Alzheimer's disease. Curcumin turns on the production of antioxidant proteins. This particular antioxidant protects the brain against oxidative injury, the culprit of aging and neurodegenerative diseases, and thus may delay the onset of the effects of aging and help prevent Alzheimer's disease when consumed often.

Cumin: Cooking with ground cumin can help prevent iron deficiency, since each teaspoon provides 4 milligrams of iron, or 22 percent of the daily recommended value. The iron found in cumin helps increase energy and is necessary to support proper metabolism for muscles and other active organs. Almost all of the cells in our body burn dietary calories to create energy through a process that requires iron.

Paprika: A small amount of paprika delivers antioxidants and nutrients. One teaspoon of paprika has 4 percent of the recommended daily intake of vitamin B6. Like most B vitamins, B6 is a coenzyme. These enzymes initiate biochemical reactions responsible for the creation of energy.

Turmeric: The yellow pigment in turmeric is called curcumin. When used regularly, curcumin helps treat diseases such as arthritis, in which free radicals are responsible for joint inflammation and damage to the joints. The combination of turmeric's antioxidant and anti-inflammatory effects on the body explains why many people with joint disease find relief when using the spice regularly.

Living a Peruvian Lifestyle

While eating a healthy diet is important for wellness, food is not the only way to decrease cortisol, prevent disease, and increase longevity. The other part of the equation is lifestyle. In addition, it's important to note that a healthy diet doesn't just entail eating superfoods but also living a superfoods lifestyle. It's not just the diet but how you eat the food, prepare the food, and manage your stress and daily living.

Mindfully selecting, preparing, and eating whole foods should be as cherished as the air we breathe. Slowing down our hectic lives is equally important for a truly nourished body and spirit. Eating should be a time of relaxation, awareness, and mindfulness. In my first book, *Eating Free*, I discussed "eating with elegance," which is not only about the sensory pleasures of food but also about the mindfulness and care we apply while eating. Eating with elegance means we sit down at the table. We enjoy these relaxing moments in life that are full of our heightened and aware senses. We take time to smell the food wafting from the kitchen. We listen to the sound of chopping as we prepare the food. We take note of the vibrant colors of the fresh produce. Finally, we taste the succulent dishes that melt in our mouths. We savor the flavor and take time to eat the meal that we have prepared with love. We eat slowly, allowing ourselves to relax.

In Peru, people take two hours on average for lunch. In the United States, we typically take five to ten minutes. I understand that not everyone has two hours during a workday. Nevertheless, we can take at least twenty minutes to sit down, chew our food, and be present in the act of eating. In addition, taking at least twenty minutes to eat will allow your stomach enough time to send the message to your brain that you are satisfied and full. If you eat too quickly, your body will push you to keep eating, and you can over-eat. When people eat too fast, they never feel satisfied. Take your time when eating and savor the flavors of your nourishing food.

Going to the farmers' market is a natural, weekly event in Peru. In Peru, people shop weekly, if not daily, for perishables. While going home from work, a Peruvian will stop in the market to buy some fresh produce or protein. We understand that the daily shopping experience may not be an option in American culture. Nevertheless, you can incorporate a weekly shopping trip to the store or local farmers' market to get the food you and your family need for the week. By having a weekly trip scheduled, you can also have a weekly meal plan in order to cook and prepare your meals and snacks as often as possible. The *Whole Body Reboot* will provide you with a list of where to find Peruvian superfoods as well as sample menus to make your buying experience as easy and effortless as possible. Now that you know about the benefits of a Peruvian superfoods diet, read on to learn how to make it work for you.

Kiwicha & Purple Corn for
BLOOD PRESSURE

Avocado & Lucuma for
HEART HEALTH

Camu Camu for
NERVOUS SYSTEM PROTECTION

Maca for
SEXUAL DRIVE & HORMONE BALANCE

Aji Pepper for
METABOLISM

Quinoa, a good source of protein for
MUSCLE MAINTENANCE

Cilantro for
ANTI-FUNGAL PROPERTIES

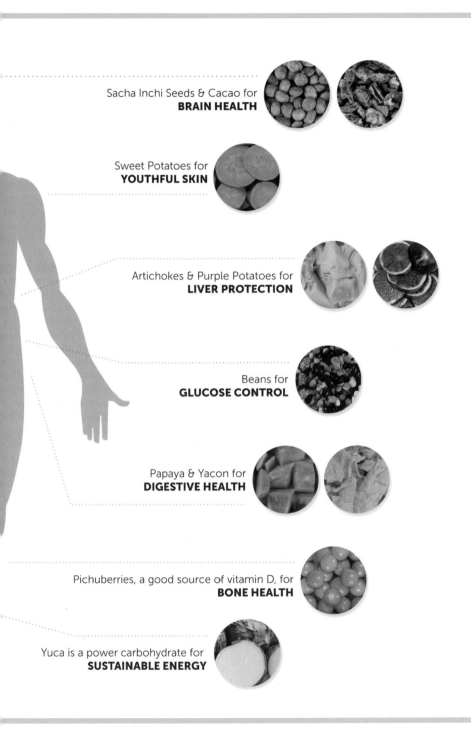

Sacha Inchi Seeds & Cacao for
BRAIN HEALTH

Sweet Potatoes for
YOUTHFUL SKIN

Artichokes & Purple Potatoes for
LIVER PROTECTION

Beans for
GLUCOSE CONTROL

Papaya & Yacon for
DIGESTIVE HEALTH

Pichuberries, a good source of vitamin D, for
BONE HEALTH

Yuca is a power carbohydrate for
SUSTAINABLE ENERGY

Superfoods by Category

Grains, starches, and legumes	Quinoa,* kiwicha, kañiwa, maca, sweet potato, purple potato, purple corn, yuca, and all beans. Other healthy options include brown rice and black rice, oatmeal, barley, and wheat berries, among others.
Fruits	Pichuberry, papaya, lucuma, camu camu, and any other fruit. Eat your colors and buy in season.
Vegetables	Artichokes, broccoli, cauliflower, Brussels sprouts, beets, asparagus, and any other vegetable. Eat your colors and buy in season.
Meats and vegetarian meats	Chicken, turkey, all white fish, salmon, eggs, tofu, tempeh, pork tenderloin, beef sirloin, or other meats with 4–7% fat.
Fats	Sacha inchi oil and seeds, olive oil, canola oil, flaxseeds, chia seeds, avocados, cacao, almonds, and walnuts, among others.
Probiotics	Yacon, Greek yogurt, kefir, tempeh, and fermented foods.
Herbs and spices	Ají, cilantro, basil, parsley, cumin, turmeric, and curry.

*Foods with purple color are from Peru.

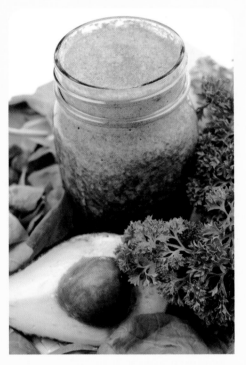

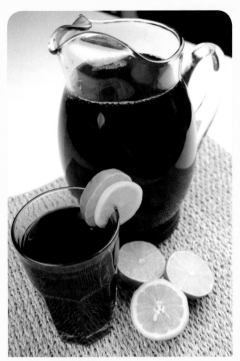

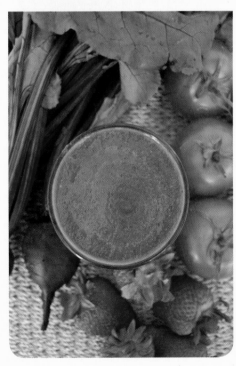

CHAPTER 2

Jump-Start Reboot Detox Plan

Starting a new program can be confusing and over-whelming. We are so accustomed to our normal habits and day-to-day routines that the thought of altering our lifestyle is daunting. You may feel stuck because you don't know how to begin. You may feel tempted by bagels at work on Wednes-days or Doughnut Fridays. You may suffer from the Weekend War-rior syndrome where you are good all week long and then blow it during the weekend fiestas. You are in a rut and don't know how to break the cycle. Therefore, your intentions to get healthy are put off for another day.

Now is the time for a brand-new kick-start. Just like when your computer freezes and you are frustrated and fed up, a simple reboot can jump-start the computer and get it working at top speed again. This week is *your* reboot. This week is meant to refresh and rebalance your internal organs. You will replenish yourself with nutrients, rejuvenate your system, and instantly revamp your health. This week will take you off the vicious cycle and prep you for your powerhouse diet plan in Chapter 3.

The Jump-Start Reboot Detox plan can be used any time of the year when you need a quick detox. For example, when you come home after a long vacation or a big holiday weekend, you may feel sluggish or out of sync. You drank too much caffeine and alcohol or you ate too many sweets and sugary treats. Basically, you ate your way through the holidays, and your clothes are squeezing the breath out of you. You suddenly notice a muffin top when wearing your skinny jeans. Now is the time to refresh, rejuvenate, and restore your health. Throughout this week you will get your balance back, realign your hormones, cleanse your internal organs, increase your energy, improve your skin, optimize your vitality, and jump-start your weight loss.

This week will begin your journey toward establishing new habits, such as planning your menu and preparing healthy meals and snacks. By setting up time for yourself and prioritizing your nutrition goals, you will set a foundation for long-term successful habits. By the end of the week, you will be motivated to continue eating delicious, nutritious foods in the days to come. **While many clients like this reboot as a way to kick-start their weight loss efforts, many others prefer to skip this detox week and move right into the regular diet plan presented in Chapter 3.** Only you can decide what works best for you.

We all should strive to eat healthy foods most days of the year, so don't be tempted to consistently overindulge and then start the Jump-Start Reboot Detox plan every Monday after a hard weekend. Weekend Warriors need to change their lifestyle habits so Mondays don't become a regular reboot day.

How the Reboot Plan Works

Each day focuses on a different color of the rainbow, like those found in the Incan flag. Every color provides a different phytonutrient, a natural chemical found in plant-based foods that prevents disease and keeps our bodies working properly. The foods also contain antioxidants that inhibit oxidation and that can protect our bodies from harmful substances such as free radicals. Because every color provides a different phytonutrient and antioxidant, you will be eating each color throughout the week so that your body reaps the benefits of optimal health.

The following colors are used in the smoothie recipes that follow:

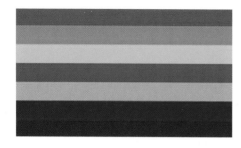

Red: Day 1

Orange: Day 2

Yellow: Day 3

Green: Day 4

Blue/Purple: Day 5

The smoothie recipes below are specifically designed for your reboot plan; every smoothie contains important micronutrients and phytochemicals to keep you balanced, nourished, and fueled. For this reboot plan, try to stick with the exact recipes provided. However, in the future, for regular daily living, you can substitute different fruits and vegetables with the same color and still reap all the benefits. For example, a client of mine detests carrots. She wouldn't touch a carrot with a ten-foot pole. Instead, she eats other orange-colored vegetables such as butternut squash and sweet potatoes. All three vegetables contain beta-carotene, which is the carotenoid found in the orange pigment. She's reaping the same benefits while enjoying her food. So take note that if you come across a particular fruit or vegetable that doesn't sound too appetizing, you're in luck! All you need to do is choose another fruit or vegetable of the same color and substitute it to ensure you keep up your optimal health. Refer to the table on page 289 to view the color swaps of different vegetables and fruits.

Each day you will be required to make three servings of the smoothie. You have two options:

Option 1: Make all three servings at once in order to save time during the day. You will need a blender that holds seven to eight cups or more in order to make three servings of the smoothie. If you do not have a blender this size, you can make the smoothie in two separate batches. Divide the smoothie into three separate mason jars to drink for your three meals of breakfast, lunch, and dinner.

Option 2: Make single-serving smoothies at different times of the day and drink for breakfast, lunch, and dinner. (We've provided you with recipes for one serving and three servings; see page 26.)

Components of the Jump-Start Reboot Detox Plan

You will drink one smoothie for breakfast, lunch, and dinner for five days. The smoothies provide you with a complete meal, including protein, carbohydrates, heart-healthy fats, vegetables, and fruits in every serving.

You will refrain from eating meat during this time for easier digestion and to clean out your system. Protein is still necessary and vital for wellness. We've tested the smoothies with natural rice protein, pea protein, and whey protein. All of these proteins have no added flavors in order to be as natural as possible with less refined or artificial sugars. We also chose complete proteins and organic protein powders in order to refrain from consuming toxic chemicals. You can choose which type of protein you want. The goal is to find a protein powder with 20–25g of protein per meal per serving for optimal performance. Various protein powders will have different grams. Keeping up your protein intake during the Jump-Start Reboot Detox plan is extremely important in order to maintain your lean muscle mass and ramp up your metabolism.

Coconut water has been included in all of the smoothies because it is a neutral choice for everyone. Coconut water is a clean energy source, providing electrolytes, potassium, and natural sugar. Since we are refraining from consuming dairy and animal products at this time, coconut water will provide you with a good base and liquid for your smoothies.

If you are hungry and need a little more than just the shake, see the sample menu below. You can add whole foods, minimally processed foods, and real foods to your daily menu. *However, the additional food below is not necessary.* What is required is that you eat three smoothies per day that are complete meals in one drink. Also take note that it is extremely important to eat every three to four hours in order to control your hunger, to keep sugar levels in check, and to maintain an active and strong metabolism.

Quick Tip: If you're worried about nutrients breaking down faster after having blended the smoothies, have no fear! The process of nutrient loss and breakdown of enzyme activity happens faster when the antioxidants are introduced to the air. So tightly seal up your smoothie, refrigerate it, and enjoy it later at your scheduled meals.

Jump-Start Reboot Detox Plan Sample Menus

BREAKFAST

Females: One serving of the smoothie of the day + optional ½ cup cooked plain oatmeal (just oats and water).

Males: One serving of the smoothie of the day + optional 1 cup cooked plain oatmeal (just oats and water).

SNACK *(optional)*

Depending on whether you are hungry, you may need a snack between breakfast and lunch or you may not. Keep in mind that these five days were developed to keep it simple and as clean as possible. Phase 2 will be full of flavor and variation.

Females: One apple + 12 unsalted almonds or ¼ cup dried pichuberries (golden berries) + 1 tablespoon of cacao nibs

Males: One apple + 18 unsalted almonds or ½ cup dried pichuberries (golden berries) + 2 tablespoons of cacao nibs

Females: One serving of the smoothie of the day + optional ½ cup cooked quinoa + ¼ avocado + non-starchy vegetables of choice (cooked or raw)

Males: One serving of the smoothie of the day + optional ¾ cup cooked quinoa + ¼ avocado + non-starchy vegetables of choice (cooked or raw)

SNACK *(optional)* ·

Females: One apple + 12 unsalted almonds or ¼ cup dried pichuberries (golden berries) + 1 tablespoon of cacao nibs

Males: One apple + 18 unsalted almonds or ½ cup dried pichuberries (golden berries) + 2 tablespoons of cacao nibs

DINNER ·

Females: One serving of the smoothie of the day + optional ½ cup black beans + Pichuberry Pico de Gallo (page 249) + non-starchy vegetables of choice (cooked or raw)

Males: One serving of the smoothie of the day + optional ¾ cup black beans + Pichuberry Pico de Gallo (page 249) + non-starchy vegetables of choice (cooked or raw)

Foods to INCLUDE	Foods to AVOID
Fruits, vegetables, heart-healthy fats, whole grains, beans	Caffeine, alcohol, refined sugar, processed foods, chemicals

Must-Dos

- ◆ **Drink water:** Drink about 2 liters per day.
- ◆ **Eat only what you need:** Each serving of smoothie provides you with a complete meal so you may not need

the additional food options during breakfast, lunch, and dinner. Refrain from overeating. Now is a time to let your body relax and get rid of excess waste.

♦ **Snack mindfully:** Pay attention to portion sizes and hunger cues.

♦ **Light exercise:** Keep your workouts to a low intensity during this week. Try walking, stretching, or hatha yoga. Refrain from running, biking, spinning, hot yoga, weight lifting, and other intense exercises. You will not be consuming enough to sustain your energy in an adequate way if you are exerting a lot through vigorous exercise. You don't want to shut down your metabolism. You want to burn fat, not muscle, during this detox. So keep exercise to a minimum and at a low intensity.

Cheat Sheet

Craving caffeine: instead try noncaffeinated green tea.

Craving salt: instead try pickled and/or fermented vegetables like kimchi, pickles, sauerkraut, cauliflower, or carrots. These are all great sources of probiotics, too.

Craving sugar: instead chew on 2 tablespoons cacao nibs (only once per day).

Craving alcohol: instead drink sparkling water with a slice of lime for a fabulous mock-tail.

Craving food: instead of dying from hunger and ruining your metabolism, have two snacks per day as necessary, one snack in the morning and one snack in the afternoon in between meals.

TIPS TO
STAY ON COURSE

❶ Choose five days when you are at home to follow the plan (this can be any five consecutive days with minimal social commitments).

❷ Shop for all of the ingredients you need before starting the plan.

❸ Give yourself time to prepare the smoothies, whether it's the night before or the morning of.

❹ Remember: if you get hungry, you have additional superfood options available.

❺ Minimal exercise is recommended so you don't over-exert yourself and increase hunger levels.

Jump-Start Reboot Detox Smoothie Recipes

Now that you have learned the do's and don'ts, you are ready to start your Whole Body Reboot weight loss plan. You can start with the optional reboot smoothie plan to follow or skip to the Weight Loss Plan on page 39.

Day 1: Red Reboot

Red represents energy, strength, power, and courage, according to color psychology. Red fruits and vegetables are rich in lycopene and anthocyanins, powerful phytochemicals that possess the characteristic red pigment. Lycopene and anthocyanins are linked with:

- Reduced risk of certain cancers
- Heart, lung, and urinary tract health
- Improved memory
- Ability to ward off infection

Ingredients	1 Serving	3 Servings
Strawberries, fresh or frozen	1½ cups	4½ cups
Tomato	½ cup	1½ cups
Cooked beets	½ cup	1½ cups
Chia seeds	1 tablespoon	3 tablespoons
Camu camu powder*	1 teaspoon	1 tablespoon
Cinnamon	¼ teaspoon	¾ teaspoon
Coconut water	1 cup	3 cups
Protein powder (rice, pea, or whey)	20–25g protein	60–75g protein

*NOTE: Camu camu is a Peruvian superfood that provides therapeutic levels of vitamin C in its natural form. Refer to the Appendix on page 290 to find where to buy camu camu. If you choose not to purchase camu camu, skip this ingredient. Another great alternative to include a Peruvian superfood with camu camu is to add a shot of youthH2O (see page 43).

❶ Put all the ingredients in a blender and puree until smooth. Add tap water until the smoothie reaches the desired consistency.

NOTE: If making the smoothie the night before, the chia seeds will absorb some of the water and it could thicken the smoothie. No worries, just add more tap water the next day and shake or stir the smoothie to the desired consistency.

Per Serving: Kcal 349, Protein 31g, Carb 48g, Fat 5g, Sodium 327mg, Dietary Fiber 15g
Daily Value: Fiber 58%, Vit C 1429%, Vit A 18%, Vit D 0%, Calcium 20%, Iron 47%

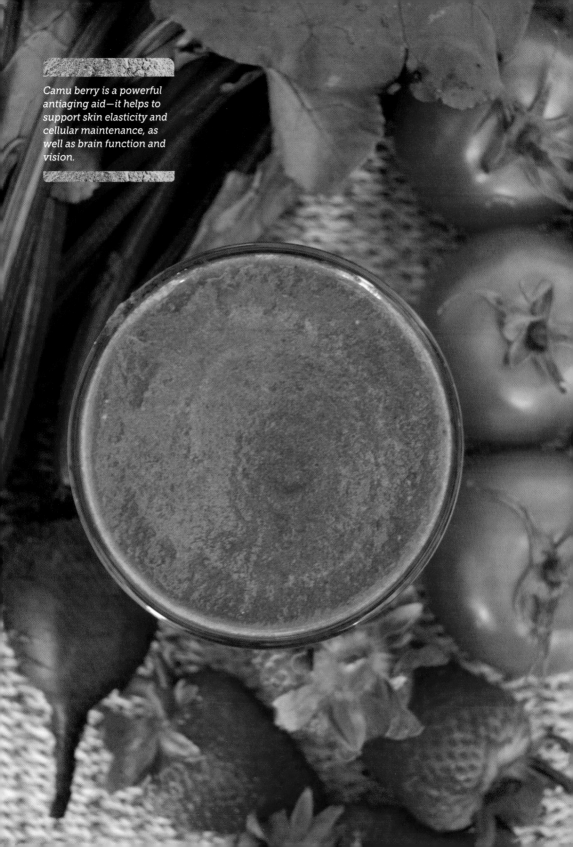

Camu berry is a powerful antiaging aid—it helps to support skin elasticity and cellular maintenance, as well as brain function and vision.

Day 2: Orange Reboot

In color theory, orange represents enthusiasm, happiness, creativity, determination, and success. Orange fruits and vegetables are loaded with carotenoids and bioflavonoids that function as antioxidants. Orange foods are also associated with high levels of vitamin C. These phytonutrients help to:

♦ Maintain a healthy immune system

♦ Slow the aging process

♦ Lower the risk of heart disease

♦ Protect against cancer

♦ Improve and maintain eye health

Ingredients	1 Serving	3 Servings
Carrots, fresh, chopped	⅓ cup	1 cup
Orange, fresh, chopped	⅓ of the fruit	1 whole fruit
Papaya, fresh, chopped	1 cup	3 cups
Coconut water	1½ cups	4½ cups
Cinnamon, ground	1 teaspoon	1 tablespoon
Chia seeds	1 tablespoon	3 tablespoons
Protein powder (rice, pea, or whey)	20–25g protein	60–75g protein

NOTE: Another great alternative to include Peruvian superfoods is to add a shot of youthH2O (see page 43).

❶ Put all the ingredients in a blender and puree until smooth. Add tap water until the smoothie is the desired consistency.

NOTE: If making the smoothie the night before, please note that the chia seeds will absorb some of the water and it could thicken the smoothie. No worries, just add more tap water the next day and shake or stir the smoothie to the desired consistency.

Per Serving: Kcal 333, Protein 30g, Carb 46g, Fat 5g, Sodium 427mg, Dietary Fiber 15g
Daily Value: Fiber 59%, Vit C 210%, Vit A 237%, Vit D 0%, Calcium 26%, Iron 34%

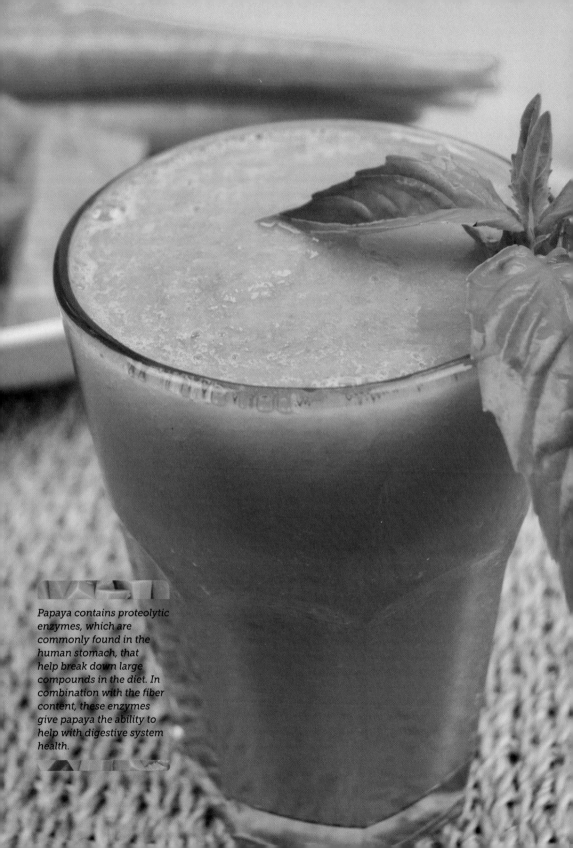

Papaya contains proteolytic enzymes, which are commonly found in the human stomach, that help break down large compounds in the diet. In combination with the fiber content, these enzymes give papaya the ability to help with digestive system health.

Day 3: Yellow Reboot

Yellow represents sunshine, happiness, intellect, and optimism, according to color theory. Yellow fruits and vegetables are rich in phytochemicals, carotenoids, and bioflavonoids. These nutrients, along with vitamin C, act as strong antioxidants. Yellow foods function to:

♦ Preserve healthy vision

♦ Maintain healthy skin and speed up wound healing

♦ Aid in heart health

♦ Boost immunity

♦ Scavenge free radicals and act as antiaging agents

Ingredients	1 Serving	3 Servings
Yellow cherry tomatoes	½ cup	1½ cups
Pichuberries*	1 cup	3 cups
Yellow squash, fresh, with skin on, chopped	½ cup	1½ cups
Pineapple	½ cup	1½ cups
Coconut water	1 cup	3 cups
Chia seeds	1 tablespoon	3 tablespoons
Turmeric	½ teaspoon	1½ teaspoons
Protein powder (rice, pea, or whey)	20–25g protein	60–75g protein

*NOTE: Pichuberries, the superfood in the smoothie, will increase your levels of vitamin D and antioxidant activity. If you can't find pichuberries, add an additional ½ cup of cherry tomatoes and ½ cup of pineapple per serving to the recipe. Another great alternative to include Peruvian superfoods is to add a shot of youthH2O (see page 43).

❶ Put all the ingredients in a blender and puree until smooth. Add tap water until the smoothie is the desired consistency.

NOTE: If making the smoothie the night before, please note that the chia seeds will absorb some of the water and it could thicken the smoothie. No worries, just add more tap water the next day and shake or stir the smoothie to the desired consistency.

Per Serving: Kcal 369, Protein 32g, Carb 53g, Fat 5g, Sodium 340mg, Dietary Fiber 11g
Daily Value: Fiber 48%, Vit C 394%, Vit A 54%, Vit D 52%, Calcium 18%, Iron 34%

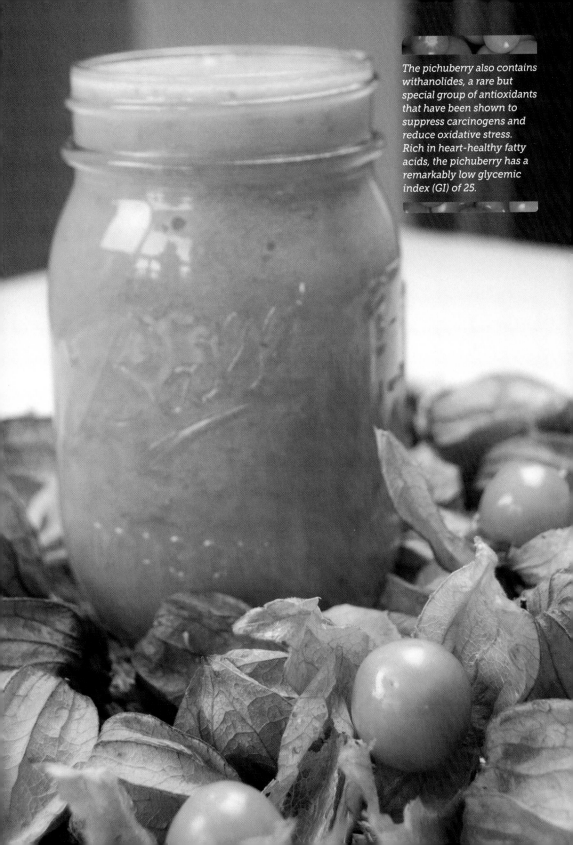

The pichuberry also contains withanolides, a rare but special group of antioxidants that have been shown to suppress carcinogens and reduce oxidative stress. Rich in heart-healthy fatty acids, the pichuberry has a remarkably low glycemic index (GI) of 25.

Day 4: Green Reboot

Green is the color of nature and represents growth, freshness, and fertility. Green fruits and vegetables are rich in lutein, zeaxanthin, and indoles. Green foods help to boost your immune system and protect against cellular damage. These phytonutrients are known for their ability to:

♦ Prevent age-related macular degeneration and cataracts

♦ Increase the rate of breakdown of carcinogens in the body

♦ Strengthen bones and teeth

Ingredients	1 Serving	3 Servings
Spinach	1 cup	3 cups
Kale	1 cup	3 cups
Cubed pineapple	½ cup	1½ cups
Chopped parsley	¼ cup	¾ cup
Avocado	⅓ of the fruit	1 whole fruit
Fresh ginger, peeled	½-inch nub	1½-inch nub
Lucuma powder*	1 tablespoon	3 tablespoons
Coconut water	1½ cups	4½ cups
Protein powder (rice, pea, or whey)	20–25g protein	60–75g protein

*NOTE: Lucuma powder is a Peruvian superfood that will provide you with many benefits. Refer to the Appendix on page 290 to find where to buy it. If you choose not to purchase lucuma, you will still get the benefits from the other ingredients. Another great alternative to include a Peruvian superfoods is to add a shot of youthH2O (see page 43).

❶ Put all the ingredients in a blender and puree until smooth. Add tap water until the smoothie is the desired consistency.

Per Serving: Kcal 388, Protein 32g, Carb 51g, Fat 8g, Sodium 449mg, Dietary Fiber 11g
Daily Value: Fiber 43%, Vit C 264%, Vit A 234%, Vit D 0%, Calcium 24%, Iron 42%

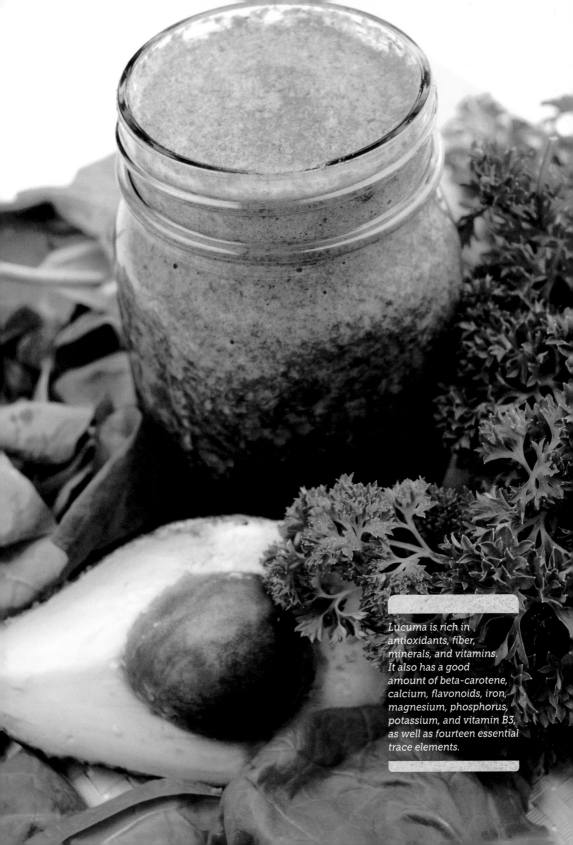

Lucuma is rich in antioxidants, fiber, minerals, and vitamins. It also has a good amount of beta-carotene, calcium, flavonoids, iron, magnesium, phosphorus, potassium, and vitamin B3, as well as fourteen essential trace elements.

Day 5: Blue/Purple Reboot

Blue is the color of peace and serenity while purple represents royalty, power, nobility, and luxury. Blue/purple fruits and vegetables aren't as numerous as some of the others; however, they are packed full of anthocyanins, phenolics, and resveratrol. These blue/purple phytonutrients have been known to:

♦ Reduce the risk of certain cancers

♦ Lower the occurrence of stroke and heart disease

♦ Improve memory function

♦ Promote healthy aging

Ingredients	1 Serving	3 Servings
Yellow squash, fresh with skin on, chopped	½ cup	1½ cups
Blueberries, fresh or frozen	¾ cup	2¼ cups
Blackberries, fresh or frozen	½ cup	1½ cups
Chicha Tisane (see page 37)*	1 cup	3 cups
Chia seeds	1 tablespoon	3 tablespoons
Protein powder (rice, pea, or whey)	20–25 g protein	60–75 g protein

*NOTE: Purple corn is the Peruvian superfood in the smoothie. Refer to the Appendix on page 290 for where to buy purple corn. If you choose not to buy purple corn, use equal parts coconut water per serving to provide enough liquid for the smoothie. Another great alternative to include a Peruvian superfood with purple corn is to add a shot of youthH2O (see page 43).

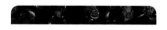

Purple corn is rich in phytonutrients called anthocyanins, which protect the body from environmental stress and toxins, strengthen the body's immunity, and protect against carcinogens. It has the highest antioxidant rating of any food, including blueberries, making it a most exciting new superfood.

1 Put all the ingredients in a blender and puree until smooth. Add tap water until the smoothie reaches the desired consistency.

NOTE: If making the smoothie the night before, the chia seeds will absorb some of the water and it could thicken the smoothie. Just add more tap water the next day and shake or stir the smoothie to the desired consistency.

Per Serving: Kcal 275, Protein 29g, Carb 33g, Fat 5g, Sodium 14mg, Dietary Fiber 12g
Daily Value: Fiber 46%, Vit C 52%, Vit A 5%, Vit D 0%, Calcium 13%, Iron 28%

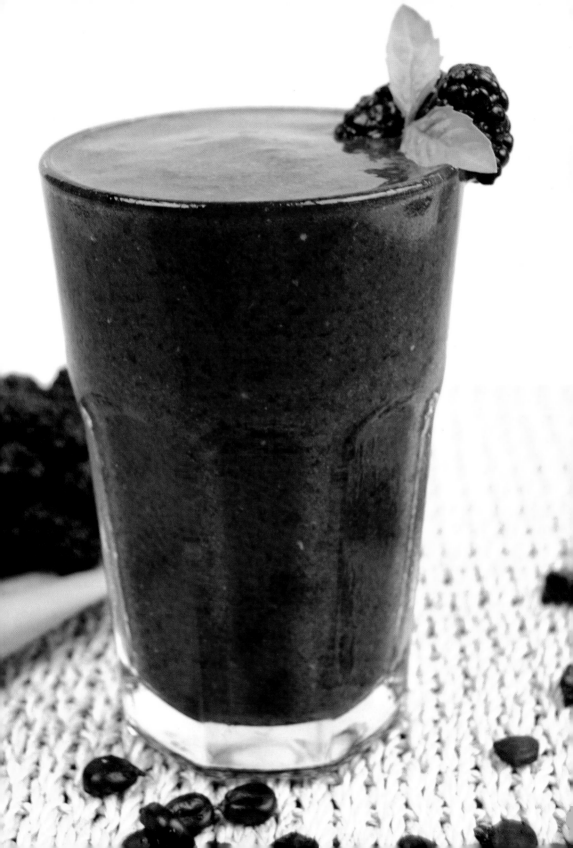

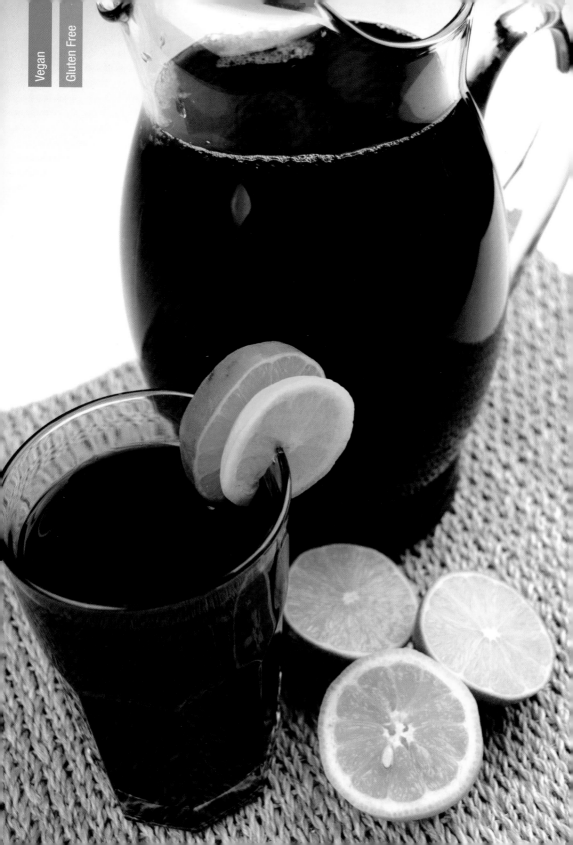

CHICHA TISANE

Prepare this drink on the weekend so you have lunch ready to go throughout the week.

❶ Put all the ingredients in a large stockpot. Bring to a boil over high heat, then lower the heat to a simmer. Cover and simmer for 45 minutes.

❷ Strain the liquid through a colander or sieve into a large container. Cool to room temperature and then refrigerate until cold.

NOTE: The tisane may be stored in the refrigerator for one to two weeks.

1 pound dried purple corn kernels

3 cinnamon sticks

1 tablespoon whole cloves

Peel of 1 pineapple (optional)

16 cups water

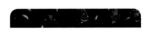

Purple corn is rich in phytonutrients, which protect the body from the environment, strengthen the body's immunity, and protect against carcinogens.

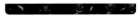

Per Serving: Kcal 68, *macronutrient content too minimal to count

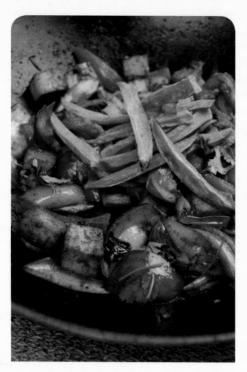

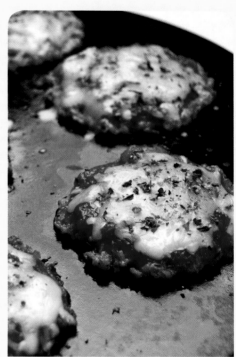

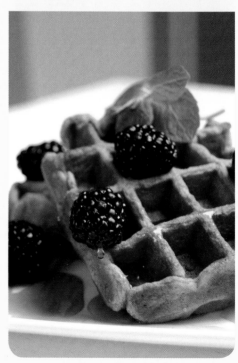

CHAPTER 3

Whole Body **Reboot** Weight Loss Plan

Many of you have finished the Jump-Start Reboot Detox plan and are feeling lighter, happier, and healthier. A lot of my clients express how they rapidly lose weight, banish bloating, and absolutely love the taste of all the fruits and vegetables so that they want to keep on drinking the smoothies. For this reason, I have devised two different plans to achieve basically the same results. One plan allows you to incorporate smoothies; the other offers a bit more variety.

Whole Body Reboot Option 1

Option I recommends you drink one or two smoothies per day and choose one or two sensible meals at either breakfast, lunch, or dinner. To learn what a sensible meal is, check out the sample menus later in the chapter according to your dietary preference. Choose a meal that sounds amazing to you and enjoy it. In addition, we all have our preferred tastes for certain smoothies. You can choose your favorite colored smoothie and repeat it for two or three days before moving on to the next color. I still recommend eating all the colors of the rainbow to obtain the various benefits so rotate your smoothies. Last of all, you will find guidelines regarding must-dos, exercise, dining out, and alcohol so read on.

Whole Body Reboot Option 2

For those of you who did not do the detox plan and are just jumping in, you will still benefit greatly from the Whole Body Reboot weight loss plan. The weight loss plan includes sample menus to help you incorporate the 21 superfoods into your daily diet. The best part about the menus is that you have multiple options and a ton of variety. For example, each menu offers seven different days where you can mix and match the various recipes for breakfast, lunch, or dinner. Not interested in making a particular recipe? No worries! Simply use another recipe from any day of the week. All of our recipes are less than 400 calories per meal, so swapping one recipe for another is completely acceptable.

To Snack or Not to Snack?

We've provided you with two to three snacks a day. If you're not hungry, you don't need to eat every single snack. The snacks are suggested in order to control hunger levels and ensure optimal energy and brain function. The main goal is to stay fueled. By eating every three to four hours, you will control ghrelin levels, which is your hunger hormone. Ghrelin spikes when we wait more than three hours between meals or skip them. Research tells us that eating every three hours is about the right interval to manage ghrelin, which controls both hunger and appetite. For example, within thirty minutes after a meal, ghrelin begins to rise steadily until the next meal. Studies have shown that a longer break between meals is associated with a more significant increase in ghrelin production. Studies have also demonstrated that there is less ghrelin produced in the average person between breakfast and lunch (a three- to four-hour break) than between lunch and dinner (typically six hours), so timing the space between meals is a critical modulator of ghrelin. With this knowledge, you may not need a snack between breakfast and lunch. But you will definitely need a snack between lunch and dinner. This is super important for controlling your hunger.

Ghrelin spikes when we lose weight. Why? Because your body only cares about survival. It wants homeostasis, or the status quo. Your body thinks losing weight is dangerous, so as you start to lose, you need to be extra mindful of your ghrelin function. Your body will fight back if you don't approach weight loss in a steady, sensible way, working with your ghrelin instead of against it. This is a fundamental principle to understand: you have to eat regularly to lose weight.

Two problems that occur during weight loss are consuming too few calories at each meal or avoiding carbohydrates. You will not have to worry about these challenges. Every meal provides you with a well-balanced mix of healthy carbohydrates, proteins, and fats in addition to adequate calorie intake.

You can approach the daily menus in many different ways. One way is to choose one day's menus and repeat that day's menus multiple times. Another way is to follow the entire sample menu exactly by cooking and prepping every meal and snack. A third way is to mix and match various breakfasts, lunches, and dinners, because the calories for each meal are roughly the same. A final way is to pick a few of your favorite meals, cook them, and eat them throughout the week. Leftovers rock! All the main dishes are filling, delicious, and nutritious. They help satisfy your hunger, control your ghrelin, and make you happier. We've provided you with four different seven-day sample menus based on your food preferences.

Sample Menu Options

We've provided a complete week of menus for "regular eaters" or those who have no dietary restrictions and eat all forms of protein and carbohydrates. However, make sure to explore and look at the other menus, too, as we've provided menus for vegans, and vegetarians, as well as gluten-free options. The various menus provide a well-balanced combination of protein, carbs, and fats using whole foods. For example, you'll find potatoes in the gluten-free menu. You can eat those, too. So check out every menu. You'll be surprised at how enticing all the recipes are.

Five Whole Body Reboot Must-Dos

The following five principles will reboot your metabolism and increase your body's energy and efficiency to burn fat and lose weight.

Reboot Must-Do #1

Eat breakfast within an hour of waking. Be sure your breakfast is a blend of carbohydrates, fiber, and protein. Our plan will offer you many recipes that satisfy this principle. Breakfast is the most important meal, and it drives your entire day. It determines how much you're going to eat at 4:00 PM. Breakfast will control ghrelin and set you up for success. If you exercise in the morning, have a pre-exercise shake (see the maca shake recipe on page 55) and then breakfast after the workout. Eating before the workout will increase your metabolism, boost your performance, help with clear thinking, improve alertness and concentration, enhance memory, and improve cognitive abilities for the entire day.

Reboot Must-Do #2

Do not skip meals. There is a lot of contradictory research about mealtimes. Some people say you should eat three meals a day, while others say you should eat five or six. For many people, three square meals don't work anymore. These days, many of us wake up at 5:00 AM and stay up until midnight. Plus, we work harder and expend more brain power, which uses up fuel. You need to eat every three to four hours to control ghrelin, so depending on how many waking hours you have, you may need four meals or you may need six.

Reboot Must-Do #3

At every meal combine carbohydrates, proteins, and fats. This gives you the optimal blend of nutritional elements to fight cravings, control hunger, and gain energy. Protein increases your metabolism while carbs lower ghrelin, help with brain function, and decrease cravings. Fat provides satiety. Every meal in the sample menus provides this optimum combination.

Reboot Must-Do #4

It doesn't matter what time you stop eating. It is a myth that we shouldn't eat after a certain time in the evening. Just give yourself at least ninety minutes before you plan to go to sleep. You need those ninety minutes to digest so you can sleep comfortably. I like to think of this as the 70/30 Rule, which means you should eat 70 percent of your calories before dinnertime and 30 percent at dinner, whatever time that may be.

Reboot Must-Do #5

Stay hydrated. You've heard it a million times, but drinking water is essential for keeping energy up, aiding metabolism, burning fat, and more. It's the fluid your body needs for life, and it's an instrumental part in your weight loss. Other fluids can be useful, but water is the best choice as it is calorie free. Forget about that whole eight cups a day thing. I want you to relax and remember to have a healthy amount of water whenever you think of it. Thirst can confuse your sense of hunger, so make sure you stay hydrated. Try infusing your water by adding pineapple or kiwi slices to it in order to provide some flavor. Make sure you throw out the pineapple or kiwi after two days and replenish it with a new batch to maintain optimal freshness.

Chicha Tisane: Optional Fluids with Power to Quench Your Thirst

Every meal plan includes Chicha Tisane (see page 37), which has more antioxidants than blueberries, making it one of the most exciting new superfoods. In addition, Chicha Tisane provides you with a flavorful alternative to plain water while helping with weight loss due to its effects on controlling blood sugar levels.

Optional Beauty and Health Enhancer

In my search for Peruvian superfoods on the market today, I came across youthH2O. YouthH2O is an age-defying supplement containing three powerful superfoods: camu camu, maca, and purple corn extract.

If you can't find purple corn, you can substitute green tea. Green tea is another fluid rich in antioxidants that will keep you hydrated during the week.

Studies have shown that maca nourishes the pituitary gland, which regulates the body's aging process. The pituitary gland is also responsible for producing somatotropin, known as HGH, which has been called the fountain of youth and has been clinically studied for its antiaging benefits.

Camu camu has a high concentration of vitamin C, which repairs and produces collagen, giving the skin a healthy, fabulous glow.

Purple corn contains the highest naturally found anthocyanin content on the planet, which aids in the prevention of heart disease, diabetes, and obesity.

We recommend adding one shot of youthH2O per day to one of your smoothies during your Jump-Start Detox Reboot week, and after the Jump-Start Reboot Detox week is over, continue to add one shot of youthH2O to one drink daily, or drink it as is for optimal vitality and benefits for at least two additional weeks. Do this for five days each week. If you skip the Jump-Start Reboot Detox week, then just add one shot of youthH2O to one drink daily or drink it as is for optimal vitality and benefits for at least three weeks. Do this for five days each week.

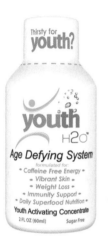

Key Points to Remember

- **Eat more whole foods and less processed foods.**
- **Frequently use heavy plant-based foods.**
- **Use more lean meats (for regular and gluten-free).**
- **Limit your red meat consumption to two servings or less than 4 ounces of red meat each week.**
- **Eat more heart-healthy fats from omega-3s and monounsaturated fats.**
- **Season your food with lots of herbs and spices.**
- **Eat healthy power carbohydrates like fruits, grains, and starches.**

- Include probiotic foods.
- Cook more at home with at least 80 percent of your meals being homemade.

Whole Body Reboot *Warmi* (Female) Weight Loss Plan

Warmi means *female* in the ancient Incan Quechua language. For women, we have chosen a caloric range of 1,300 calories to lose weight. This plan was developed for females who are twenty to fifty-nine years old, with an average lifestyle including a desk job. During the weight loss phase, we recommend weekly exercise. Refer to the Whole Body Reboot Exercise plan (page 54) for specific recommendations. For women older than sixty years old who exercise three times or less per week, you will need to cut your calories by 100 per day in order to successfully lose weight. As we age gracefully, our metabolisms naturally decrease. Therefore, by eliminating one snack every day from the sample menus, you can cut the extra 100 calories you do not need for optimal weight loss. Another option is to adjust your lunch or dinner by reducing your portion size slightly. For example, eat 50 calories less at lunch and at dinner. Simply cut 50 calories by reducing your carbohydrate intake by half.

Whole Body Reboot *Qhari* (Male) Weight Loss Plan

Qhari means *male* in the ancient Incan Quechua language. For men, we have chosen a caloric range of 1,800 calories to lose weight. This plan was developed for males from twenty to sixty-nine years old, with an average lifestyle including a desk job. During the weight loss phase, we recommend weekly exercise. Refer to the Whole Body Reboot Exercise plan (page 54) for specific recommendations.

REGULAR 1300 CALORIE 7-DAY MENU

	MONDAY	TUESDAY	WEDNESDAY	THURSDAY	FRIDAY	SATURDAY	SUNDAY
BREAKFAST	1 Power Morning Spinach Egg-White Omelet (p74), 1 Yuca Artichoke Patty, (p 229), 1 (3 ounce) chicken sausage	1 cup Quinoa Pumpkin Porridge (p 81), 1 cup unsweetened almond milk, 1 hardboiled egg	1 slice Purple Potato Frittata (p 77), 1 cup mixed berries	3 Quinoa, Spinach, & Egg-White Muffins (p 79), 1 cup low fat milk	2½ cups Triple Berry Breakfast Smoothie (p 156)	1½ cups Very Coconutty Kañiwa Cereal (p 96)	1 Sweet Potato Waffle (p 91), 1 cup mixed berries, 2 tablespoons yacon syrup (or 1 tablespoon agave)
SNACK	1 Inca Power Bar (p 215)	½ cup cubed papaya, ¾ cup low-fat Greek yogurt, 4 walnut halves	¼ cup Power Trail Mix (p 221)	¼ cup Avocado Hummus (p 241), 1 cup vegetable sticks	1 apple, 1 hardboiled egg	¼ cup Avocado Hummus (p 241), 1 cup vegetable sticks	⅔ cup Papaya Tropical Fruit Salad (p 177)
LUNCH	1 Mu Shu Pork–Peruvian Fusion Lettuce Cup (p 173), 1 cup Chicha Tisane (p 37)	1½ cups Sacha Inchi Salmon Salad (p 183), 1 cup Chicha Tisane (p 37)	1 Avocado Queso Fresco Sandwich (p 162), 2 cups arugula salad, 2 tablespoons lemon juice, 1 cup Chicha Tisane (p 37)	½ Chicken Avocado Wrap (p 169), ½ cup fruit salad, 1 cup Chicha Tisane (p 37)	3 cups Zesty Kale & Veggie Salad with Chicken Sausage (p 189), 1 cup Chicha Tisane (p 37)	2 cups Pichuberry Gazpacho (p 201), 4 ounces Weekend Oregano Roasted Chicken (p 152), 1 cup Chicha Tisane (p 37)	4 ounces Lemon Roasted Fish (p 119), 1 tablespoon Cilantro Chimichurri (p 244), ½ cup Choclo Chopped Salad (p 171), 1 cup Chicha Tisane (p 37)
SNACK	½ cup cubed papaya, ¾ cup low-fat Greek yogurt, 4 walnut halves	1 Inca Power Bar (p 215)	⅔ cup Papaya Tropical Fruit Salad (p 177)	¼ cup Power Trail Mix (p 221)	¼ cup Roasted Garlic Artichoke Dip (p 251), 1 ounce crackers	1 apple, 1 tablespoon sacha inchi butter (or nut butter of choice)	¼ cup Avocado Hummus (p 241), 1 cup vegetable sticks
DINNER	4.5 ounces Grilled Salmon (p 111), ½ cup black rice, 3½ cups spinach salad, ¼ cup Pichuberry Honey Mustard Dressing (p 246)	4 ounces Weekend Oregano Roasted Chicken (p 152), ½ cup Pichuberry Pico de Gallo (p 249), 2 wedges Yuca Fries (p 231)	3 cups Parihuela (Peruvian Seafood Soup) (p 199)	½ cup Choclo (large corn) (p 235), ½ Boiled Sweet Potato (p 234), 1 skewer Beef Anticuchos (p 105)	½ Grilled Shrimp-Stuffed Avocado (p 113), ½ cup Plantain Chips (p 219)	1½ cups Lomo Saltado (p 121), ½ cup Baked Sweet Potato Fries (p 213)	2 Quinoa Parmesan Pizzettes (p 135), 2 cups mixed greens, 2 tablespoons lemon juice
TREAT	1 Pineapple Lucuma Ice Pop (p 277)	1 Dark Chocolate Fig with Cacao Nibs (p 267)	3 Dark Chocolate-Covered Pichuberries (p 265)	1 tablespoon Inchi-Tella (p 273), ½ cup strawberries	1 Dark Chocolate Fig with Cacao Nibs (p 267)	1 Yummy Stuffed Date with Cacao and Walnuts (p 288)	3 Dark Chocolate-Covered Pichuberries (p 265)

REGULAR 1800 CALORIE 7-DAY MENU

	MONDAY	TUESDAY	WEDNESDAY	THURSDAY	FRIDAY	SATURDAY	SUNDAY
BREAKFAST	1 Power Morning Spinach Egg-White Omelet (p74), 1 Yuca Artichoke Patty (p 229), 1 (3 ounce) chicken sausage	1½ cups Quinoa Pumpkin Porridge (p 81), 1 cup unsweetened almond milk, 1 hardboiled egg	2 slices Purple Potato Frittata (p 77), 1 cup cubed papaya, 1 cup low-fat milk	3 Quinoa, Spinach, & Egg-White Muffins (p 79), 1 cup low fat milk	2½ cups Triple-Berry Breakfast Smoothie (p 156)	3 cups Very Coconutty Kañiwa Cereal (p 96)	2 Sweet Potato Waffles (p 91), ½ cup mixed berries, 1 tablespoon yacon syrup (or 2 teaspoons agave)
SNACK	1 Inca Power Bar (p 215)	½ cup cubed papaya, ¾ cup low-fat Greek yogurt, 4 walnut halves	¼ cup Power Trail Mix (p 221), ¾ cup low-fat Greek yogurt	¼ cup Avocado Hummus (p 241), 1 cup vegetable sticks	1 apple, ¾ cup low-fat Greek yogurt	¼ cup Avocado Hummus (p 241), 1 cup vegetable sticks	⅔ cup Papaya Tropical Fruit Salad (p 177)
LUNCH	2 Mu Shu Pork–Peruvian Fusion Lettuce Cup (p 173), 1 cup Chicha Tisane (p 37)	3 cups Sacha Inchi Salmon Salad (p 183), 1 cup Chicha Tisane (p 37)	1 Avocado Queso Fresco Sandwich (p 162), 2 cups arugula salad, 2 tablespoons lemon juice, 1 cup Chicha Tisane (p 37)	1 Chicken Avocado Wrap (p 169), 1 cup fruit salad, 1 cup Chicha Tisane (p 37)	4 cups Zesty Kale & Veggie Salad with Chicken Sausage (p 189), 1 cup Chicha Tisane (p 37)	3 cups Pichuberry Gazpacho (p 201), 4 ounces Weekend Oregano Roasted Chicken (p 152), 1 cup Chicha Tisane (p 37)	4 ounces Lemon Roasted Fish (p 119), 1 tablespoon Cilantro Chimichuri (p 244), 1 cup Choclo Chopped Salad (p 171), 1 cup Chicha Tisane (p 37)
SNACK	½ cup cubed papaya, ¾ cup low-fat Greek yogurt, 4 walnut halves	1 Inca Power Bar (p 215)	⅔ cup Papaya Tropical Fruit Salad (p 177)	⅔ cup Papaya Tropical Fruit Salad (p 177)	¼ cup Roasted Garlic Artichoke Dip (p 251), 1 ounce crackers	¾ cup berries, ¾ cup low-fat Greek yogurt	¼ cup Avocado Hummus (p 241), 1 cup vegetable sticks
DINNER	4.5 ounces Grilled Salmon (p 111), ½ cup black rice, 3½ cups spinach salad, ¼ cup Pichuberry Honey Mustard Dressing (p 246)	4 ounces Weekend Oregano Roasted Chicken (p 152), ½ cup Pichuberry Pico de Gallo (p 249), 4 wedges Yuca Fries (p 231)	4½ cups Parhuela (Peruvian Seafood Soup) (p 199)	½ cup Choclo (large corn) (p 235), ½ Boiled Sweet Potato (p 234), 2 skewers Beef Anticuchos (p 105)	1 Grilled Shrimp-Stuffed Avocado (p 113), ½ cup Plantain Chips (p 219)	1½ cups Lomo Saltado (p 121), ½ cup Baked Sweet Potato Fries (p 213)	3 Quinoa Parmesan Pizzettes (p 135), 2 cups mixed greens, 2 tablespoons lemon juice
TREAT	1 Pineapple Lucuma Ice Pop (p 277)	1 Dark Chocolate Fig with Cacao Nibs (p 267)	5 Dark Chocolate-Covered Pichuberries (p 265)	1 tablespoon Inchi-Tella (p 273), ¾ cup strawberries	1 Dark Chocolate Fig with Cacao Nibs (p 267)	1 Yummy Stuffed Date with Cacao and Walnuts (p 288)	5 Dark Chocolate-Covered Pichuberries (p 265)

GLUTEN-FREE 1300 CALORIE 7-DAY MENU

	MONDAY	TUESDAY	WEDNESDAY	THURSDAY	FRIDAY	SATURDAY	SUNDAY
BREAKFAST	1¾ cups Breakfast Brain-Food Parfait (p 62)	1 Gluten-Free Quinoa Crepe (p 67), ¼ tomato, 2 tablespoons avocado, 2 pieces turkey bacon	3 cups Chia Cacao Protein Shake (p 154)	2 cups Breakfast of Champions à la Peruvian (p 63)	1 Gluten-Free Pichuberry Scone (p 65), 1 cup unsweetened almond milk	1 Sweet Potato Waffle (p 91), ½ cup mixed berries, 1 tablespoon yacon syrup (or 2 teaspoons agave)	1½ cups Mediterranean Peruvian Fusion Scramble (p 69)
SNACK	¾ cup berries, ½ cup low-fat Greek yogurt	¼ cup Power Trail Mix (p 221)	1 Inca Power Bar (p 215)	¼ cup Roasted Garlic Artichoke Dip (p 251), 1 ounce crackers	½ cup unsweetened applesauce, 1 tablespoon chia seeds	1 Caprese Pichuberry Skewer (p 214)	1 apple, 1 tablespoon sacha inchi butter (or nut butter of choice)
LUNCH	1 Turkey Pichuberry Burger Patty (p 149), 3 wedges Yuca Fries (p 231), 1 cup Chicha Tisane (p 37)	4 ounces Weekend Oregano Roasted Chicken (p 152), 1 cup Beet & Orange Salad with Pichuberry Champagne Vinaigrette (p 163), ½ cup black rice, 1 cup Chicha Tisane (p 37)	4.5 ounces Grilled Salmon (p 111), ½ Roasted Sweet Plantain (p 232), 3½ cups mixed greens, 2 tablespoons lemon juice, 1 cup Chicha Tisane (p 37)	1 piece Tacu Tacu (p 141), 4 ounces Weekend Oregano Roasted Chicken (p 152), 3½ cups mixed greens, 2 tablespoons lemon juice, 1 cup Chicha Tisane (p 37)	1 Pulled Pork Taco (p 181), ½ cup Pichuberry Pico de Gallo (p 249), 3½ cups mixed greens, 2 tablespoons lemon juice, 1 cup Chicha Tisane (p 37)	4.5 ounces Lemon-Roasted Fish (p 119), ¾ cup Lima Bean Stew (p 195), 1 cup Chicha Tisane (p 37)	¾ cup Peruvian-Style Ceviche (p 179), ½ Boiled Sweet Potato (p 234), ½ cup Choclo (large corn) (p 235), 1 cup Chicha Tisane (p 37)
SNACK	⅔ cup Papaya Tropical Fruit Salad (p 177)	1 apple, ½ cup low-fat Greek yogurt	½ cup unsweetened applesauce, 1 tablespoon chia seeds	¼ cup Power Trail Mix (p 221)	⅔ cup Papaya Tropical Fruit Salad (p 177)	1 medium apple	1 Caprese Pichuberry Skewer (p 214)
DINNER	4.5 ounces Pork Tenderloin with Peruvian Spice Rub (p 131), ½ cup black rice, ½ cup Salsa Criolla (p 253)	1 cup Purple Potato Leek Soup (p 205), 3 ounces sirloin steak, 3½ cups mixed greens, 2 tablespoons lemon juice	1 cup Pichuberry Chicken Cacciatore (p 129), 1 cup steamed broccoli, 2 tablespoons lemon juice	1 Peruvian Fish Packet (p 125), ½ Baked Sweet Potatoes Fries with Coconut Oil (p 213)	4 ounces Weekend Oregano Roasted Chicken (p 152), ½ cup Roasted Artichoke Mashed Potatoes (p 223), ½ cup Roasted Vegetables (p 225)	1½ cups Wholesome Roasted Eggplant Stew (p 210), ½ cup Quinoa (p 238)	2 cups Chicken Tallarin Saltado (p 107)
TREAT	3 Dark Chocolate-Covered Pichuberries (p 265)	1 Yummy Stuffed Date with Cacao and Walnuts (p 288)	3 Dark Chocolate-Covered Pichuberries (p 265)	1 Dark Chocolate Fig with Cacao Nibs (p 267)	1 Strawberry Maca Frozen Yogurt Pop (p 283)	1 Stuffed Date with Cacao and Walnuts (p 288)	1 Dark Chocolate Fig with Cacao Nibs (p 267)

GLUTEN-FREE 1800 CALORIE 7-DAY MENU

	MONDAY	TUESDAY	WEDNESDAY	THURSDAY	FRIDAY	SATURDAY	SUNDAY
BREAKFAST	1¾ cups Breakfast Brain-Food Parfait (p 62)	2 Gluten-Free Quinoa Crepes (p 67), ½ tomato, ¼ cup avocado, 3 pieces turkey bacon	3 cups Chia Cacao Protein Shake (p 154)	2 cups Breakfast of Champions à la Peruvian (p 63)	1 Gluten-Free Pichuberry Scone (p 65), 1 cup unsweetened almond milk, 1 cup berries	2 Sweet Potato Waffles (p 91), ½ cup mixed berries, 2 tablespoons yacon syrup (or 2 teaspoons agave)	2½ cups Mediterranean Peruvian Fusion Scramble (p 69)
SNACK	¾ cup berries, ½ cup low-fat Greek yogurt	¼ cup Power Trail Mix (p 221)	1 Inca Power Bar (p 215)	¼ cup Roasted Garlic Artichoke Dip (p 251), 1 ounce crackers	½ cup unsweetened applesauce, 1 tablespoon chia seeds	1 Caprese Pichuberry Skewer (p 214)	1 apple, 1 tablespoon sacha inchi butter (or nut butter of choice)
LUNCH	2 Turkey Pichuberry Burger Patties (p 149), 3 wedges Yuca Fries (p 231), 1 cup Chicha Tisane (p 37)	4 ounces Weekend Oregano Roasted Chicken (p 152), 1½ cups Beet & Orange Salad with Pichuberry Champagne Vinaigrette (p 163), 1 cup black rice, 1 cup Chicha Tisane (p 37)	4.5 ounces Grilled Salmon (p 111), 1 Roasted Sweet Plantain (p 232), 3½ cups mixed greens, 2 tablespoons lemon juice, 1 cup Chicha Tisane (p 37)	2 pieces Tacu Tacu (p 141), 4 ounces Weekend Oregano Roasted Chicken (p 152), 3½ cups mixed greens, 2 tablespoons lemon juice, 1 cup Chicha Tisane (p 37)	2 Pulled Pork Tacos (p 181), ½ cup Pichuberry Pico de Gallo (p 249), 3½ cups mixed greens, 2 tablespoons lemon juice, 1 cup Chicha Tisane (p 37)	4.5 ounces Lemon-Roasted Fish (p 119), 1½ cups Lima Bean Stew (p 195), 1 cup Chicha Tisane (p 37)	1 cup Peruvian-Style Ceviche (p 179), ½ Boiled Sweet Potato (p 234), ½ cup Choclo (large corn) (p 235), 1 cup Chicha Tisane (p 37)
SNACK	⅔ cup Papaya Tropical Fruit Salad (p 177)	1 apple, ¾ cup low-fat Greek yogurt	½ cup unsweetened applesauce, 1 tablespoon chia seeds	¼ cup Power Trail Mix (p 221)	⅔ cup Papaya Tropical Fruit Salad (p 177)	1 medium apple	2 Caprese Pichuberry Skewer (p 214)
DINNER	4.5 ounces Pork Tenderloin with Peruvian Spice Rub (p 131), 1 cup black rice, ½ cup Salsa Criolla (p 253)	1 cup Purple Potato Leek Soup (p 205), 4 ounces sirloin steak, 3½ cups mixed greens, 2 tablespoons lemon juice	2 cups Pichuberry Chicken Cacciatore (p 129), 1 cup steamed broccoli, 2 tablespoons lemon juice	2 Peruvian Fish Packets (p 125), ½ Baked Sweet Potatoes Fries with Coconut Oil (p 213)	4 ounces Weekend Oregano Roasted Chicken (p 152), ½ cup Roasted Artichoke Mashed Potatoes (p 223), ½ cup Roasted Vegetables (p 225)	2 cups Wholesome Roasted Eggplant Stew (p 210), ½ cup Quinoa (p 238)	2 cups Chicken Tallarin Saltado (p 107)
TREAT	5 Dark Chocolate-Covered Pichuberries (p 265)	1 Stuffed Date with Cacao and Walnuts (p 288)	5 Dark Chocolate-Covered Pichuberries (p 265)	1 Dark Chocolate Fig with Cacao Nibs (p 267)	1 Strawberry Maca Frozen Yogurt Pop (p 283)	1 Stuffed Date with Cacao and Walnuts (p 288)	1 Dark Chocolate Fig with Cacao Nibs (p 267)

VEGAN 1300 CALORIE 7-DAY MENU

	MONDAY	TUESDAY	WEDNESDAY	THURSDAY	FRIDAY	SATURDAY	SUNDAY
BREAKFAST	¼ cup Peruvian Kiwicha Granola (p 73), ½ cup unsweetened coconut milk yogurt, ¾ cup blueberries	1 cup Savory Polenta with Curried Garbanzo and Arugula (p 85), 1 cup cubed papaya	4 cups Silky Papaya Smoothie (p 155)	1 cup Tofu Breakfast Scramble (p 93), 1 slice whole grain bread, 2 tablespoons avocado, ½ tomato	1²/₃ cups Quinoa Cranberry Coco Fusion (p 80)	1 Vegan Pichuberry Pancake (p 95), 1 tablespoon yacon syrup (or 2 teaspoons agave) Make a shake: 1 cup unsweetened almond milk, vegan protein powder (20–25g protein)	1 cup Sweet Potato Kiwicha Breakfast Bake (p 89). Make a shake: 1 cup unsweetened almond milk, vegan protein powder (20–25g protein)
SNACK	½ cup unsweetened applesauce, 1 tablespoon chia seeds	¼ cup Roasted Garlic Artichoke Dip (p 251), 1 cup vegetable sticks	1 Superfood Four-Seed Bite (p 227)	½ Boiled Sweet Potato (p 234), ½ cup unsweetened coconut milk yogurt, 4 walnut halves	¼ cup Avocado Hummus (p 241), 1 cup vegetable sticks	¼ cup Power Trail Mix (p 221)	¼ cup Peruvian Kiwicha Granola (p 73), ¾ cup unsweetened coconut milk yogurt
LUNCH	1 cup Peruvian Beans à la Cilantro (p 123), 2 slices Roasted Miso Tofu (p 257), 1 cup steamed broccoli, 1 tablespoon lemon juice, 1 cup Chicha Tisane (p 37)	2 cups Lentil-Quinoa Masachakuy (p 120), 3 cups mixed greens, 1 tablespoon balsamic vinegar, 1 cup Chicha Tisane (p 37)	4 Quinoa Canellini Bean Croquettes (p 133), 3½ cups mixed greens, 1 tablespoon balsamic vinegar, 1 cup Chicha Tisane (p 37)	½ Nori Wrap à la Peruvian (p 175), ½ cup cubed mango, 1½ cups sliced cucumber, 1 tablespoon lemon juice, 1 cup Chicha Tisane (p 37)	1²/₃ cups Andean Potato Salad (p 161), 2 slices Garlic Roasted Miso Tofu (p 237), 1 cup Chicha Tisane (p 37)	1½ cups Pichuberry Quinoa Chili (p 203), 1 cup Chicha Tisane (p 37)	1 Tempeh White Bean Ceviche Lettuce Cup (p 185), 1 cup Chicha Tisane (p 37)
SNACK	¼ cup Power Trail Mix (p 221)	1 Superfood Four-Seed Bite (p 227)	½ Boiled Sweet Potato (p 234), ½ cup unsweetened coconut milk yogurt, 4 walnut halves	½ cup unsweetened applesauce, 1 tablespoon chia seeds	Make a shake: 1 cup unsweetened almond milk, vegan protein powder (20–25g protein), ¾ cup blueberries	¼ cup Avocado Hummus (p 241), 1 cup vegetable sticks	¼ cup Roasted Garlic Artichoke Dip (p 251), 1 cup vegetable sticks
DINNER	2 slices Kiwicha Crusted Tempeh (p 117), ¼ cup Avocado Mango Salsa (p 242), 3 cups mixed greens, 2 tablespoons lemon juice	2 cups Estofado de Seitan (p 193)	¼ recipe Roasted Spaghetti Squash Primavera (p 139), 2 slices Garlic Roasted Miso Tofu (p 237)	½ Quinoa-Stuffed Bell Pepper (p 137), 1 cup Roasted Vegetables (p 225)	1 cup Tofu Saltado (p 147), 1 cup black rice	1 Veggie Causa with Tofu (p 151), 2 tablespoons Aji Vinaigrette (p 240)	2 Peruvian Spiced Seitan and Veggie Shish Kebabs (p 127), 2 Yuca Fries (p 231)
TREAT	2 Popped Kiwicha Chocolate Medallions (p 279)	½ cup Lucuma Pudding (p 274)	2 Popped Kiwicha Chocolate Medallions (p 279)	1 Pichuberry Pineapple Skewer (p 275)	3 Dark Chocolate–Covered Pichuberries (p 265)	½ Baked Apple with Cinnamon and Chia (p 259)	3 Dark Chocolate–Covered Pichuberries (p 265)

VEGAN 1800 CALORIE 7-DAY MENU

	MONDAY	TUESDAY	WEDNESDAY	THURSDAY	FRIDAY	SATURDAY	SUNDAY
BREAKFAST	¼ cup Peruvian Kiwicha Granola (p 73), ¾ cup unsweetened coconut milk yogurt, ¾ cup blueberries	1½ cups Savory Polenta with Curried Garbanzo and Arugula (p 85), 1 cup cubed papaya	4 cups Silky Papaya Smoothie (p 155)	1 cup Tofu Breakfast Scramble (p 93), 1 slice whole grain bread, ¼ cup avocado, ½ tomato. Make a shake: 1 cup unsweetened almond milk, vegan protein powder (20–25g protein)	2 cups Quinoa Cranberry Coco Fusion (p 80)	2 Vegan Pichuberry Pancakes (p 95), 1½ tablespoons yacon syrup (or 2 teaspoons agave) Make a shake: 1 cup unsweetened almond milk, vegan protein powder (20–25g protein)	1½ cups Sweet Potato Kiwicha Breakfast Bake (p 89). Make a shake: 1 cup unsweetened almond milk, vegan protein powder (20–25g protein)
SNACK	¾ cup unsweetened applesauce, 1 tablespoon chia seeds	½ cup Roasted Garlic Artichoke Dip (p 251), 1 cup vegetable sticks	2 Superfood Four-Seed Bites (p 227)	½ Boiled Sweet Potato (p 234), ¾ cup unsweetened coconut milk yogurt, 4 walnut halves	½ cup Avocado Hummus (p 241), 1 cup vegetable sticks	¼ cup Power Trail Mix (p 221)	¼ cup Peruvian Kiwicha Granola (p 73), ¾ cup unsweetened coconut milk yogurt
LUNCH	1½ cups Peruvian Beans à la Cilantro (p 123), 3 slices Garlic Roasted Miso Tofu (p 237), 1 cup steamed broccoli, 1 tablespoon lemon juice, 1 cup Chicha Tisane (p 37)	2½ cups Lentil-Quinoa Masachakuy (p 120), 3 cups mixed greens, 1 tablespoon balsamic vinegar, 1 cup Chicha Tisane (p 37)	6 Quinoa Canellini Bean Croquettes (p 133), 3½ cups mixed greens, 1 tablespoon balsamic vinegar, 1 cup Chicha Tisane (p 37)	1 Nori Wrap à la Peruvian (p 175), ½ cup cubed mango, 1½ cups sliced cucumber, 1 tablespoon lemon juice, 1 cup Chicha Tisane (p 37)	1⅔ cups Andean Potato Salad (p 161), 3 slices Garlic Roasted Miso Tofu (p 237), 1 cup Chicha Tisane (p 37)	2 cups Pichuberry Quinoa Chili (p 203), 1 cup Chicha Tisane (p 37)	2 Tempeh White Bean Ceviche Lettuce Cups (p 185), 1 medium apple, 1 cup Chicha Tisane (p 37)
SNACK	¼ cup Power Trail Mix (p 221), 1 cup cubed papaya	2 Superfood Four-Seed Bites (p 227), 1 medium apple	½ Boiled Sweet Potato (p 234), ¾ cup unsweetened coconut milk yogurt, 4 walnut halves	½ cup unsweetened applesauce, 1 tablespoon chia seeds	Make a shake: 1 cup unsweetened almond milk, vegan protein powder (20–25g protein), ¾ cup blueberries	¼ cup Avocado Hummus (p 241), 1 cup vegetable sticks	¼ cup Roasted Garlic Artichoke Dip (p 251), 1 cup vegetable sticks
DINNER	3 slices Kiwicha Crusted Tempeh (p 117), ½ cup Avocado Mango Salsa (p 242), 3 cups mixed greens, 2 tablespoons lemon juice	2 cups Estofado de Seitan (p 193)	¼ recipe Roasted Spaghetti Squash Primavera (p 139), 3 slices Garlic Roasted Miso Tofu (p 237)	½ Quinoa-Stuffed Bell Pepper (p 137), 1½ cups Roasted Vegetables (p 225)	1½ cups Tofu Saltado (p 147), ½ cup black rice	1 Veggie Causa with Tofu (p 151), 2 tablespoons Aji Vinaigrette (p 240)	3 Peruvian Spiced Seitan and Veggie Shish Kebabs (p 127), 3 Yuca Fries (p 251)
TREAT	2 Popped Kiwicha Chocolate Medallions (p 279)	½ cup Lucuma Pudding (p 274)	1 Yummy Stuffed Date with Cacao and Walnuts (p 288)	2 Pichuberry Pineapple Skewers (p 275)	2 Popped Kiwicha Chocolate Medallions (p 279)	1 Baked Apple with Cinnamon and Chia (p 259)	½ cup Lucuma Pudding (p 274)

VEGETARIAN 1300 CALORIE 7-DAY MENU

	MONDAY	TUESDAY	WEDNESDAY	THURSDAY	FRIDAY	SATURDAY	SUNDAY
BREAKFAST	¼ cup Oven-Roasted Pichuberries (p 217), 6 egg whites (¾ cup), scrambled, 1 slice whole grain bread, toasted	1 cup Sweet Potato Crustless Quiche (p 87), 1 cup cubed papaya	1 tablespoon Pichuberry Marmalade (p 247), 1 slice whole grain bread, toasted, 2 ounces skim queso fresco cheese	2 cups Power-Packed Incan Parfait (p 75)	1 Quinoa Pichuberry Muffin (p 83), 6 egg whites (¾ cup), scrambled, ½ cup salsa	Make a shake: 1 cup unsweetened almond milk, 1 cup berries, vegetarian protein powder (20–25g protein), 1 tablespoon chia seeds	1 slice Overnight Lucuma French Toast (p 71), 1 tablespoon yacon syrup (or 2 teaspoons agave)
SNACK	¼ cup Avocado Hummus (p 241), 1 cup vegetable sticks	Make a shake: 1 cup unsweetened almond milk, ¾ cup berries, vegetarian protein powder (20–25g protein)	¼ cup Power Trail Mix (p 221)	1 Inca Power Bar (p 215)	¾ cup berries, ½ cup low-fat Greek yogurt	½ cup unsweetened applesauce, 1 tablespoon chia seeds	¼ cup Roasted Garlic Artichoke Dip (p 251), 1 cup vegetable sticks
LUNCH	1 White Bean Avocado Wrap (p 187), 3½ cups mixed greens, 2 tablespoons lemon juice, 1 cup Chicha Tisane (p 37)	1 cup Garbanzo Saltado (p 109), 6 cups raw spinach, steamed, 1 tablespoon lemon juice, 1 cup Chicha Tisane (p 37)	2 skewers Tofu à la Panca (p 145), ½ cup black beans, 3½ cups mixed greens, 2 tablespoons lemon juice, 1 cup Chicha Tisane (p 37)	2 cups Minestrone with Quinoa Noodles (p 197), 3½ cups mixed greens, 2 tablespoons lemon juice, 1 cup Chicha Tisane (p 37)	2 Black Bean & Sweet Potato Thai Fusion Tacos (p 165), 1 cup Chicha Tisane (p 37)	1½ cups Butternut Squash & Legumes Quinoa Salad (p 167), 2 tablespoons Cucumber-Cilantro Lime Dressing (p 245), 1 cup Chicha Tisane (p 37)	1 cup Zesty Vegan Chickpea Salad (p 190), ½ whole grain pita bread, 1 cup lettuce, ¼ cup tomato, 1 cup Chicha Tisane (p 37)
SNACK	½ Boiled Sweet Potato (p 234), ¼ cup low-fat Greek yogurt, 4 walnut halves	½ cup unsweetened applesauce, 1 tablespoon chia seeds	1 medium apple, 1 hard-boiled egg	¼ cup Roasted Garlic Artichoke Dip (p 251), 1 ounce crackers	1 Inca Power Bar (p 215)	¼ cup Avocado Hummus (p 241), 1 cup vegetable sticks	¼ cup Power Trail Mix (p 221)
DINNER	1½ cups Arroz con Tofu (p 101), ¼ cup Salsa Criolla (p 253)	2 slices Tempeh Milanese (p 143), ½ cup cooked pasta, ½ cup marinara sauce	1 cup Trigo Guisado (p 209), 1 cup cooked broccoli, 2 tablespoons lemon juice	1 cup Garlic Butter Beans à la Parmesan (p 110), 1 (3 ounce) vegetarian sausage	1½ cups Tofu Vegetable Aji Panca Curry (p 207), ½ cup black rice	1 cup Aji de Tempeh (p 98), 1 cup cooked zucchini, 1 hard-boiled egg	1 cup Artichoke Seitan Molido (p 103), ½ cup brown rice
TREAT	3 Dark Chocolate–Covered Pichuberries (p 265)	½ cup Citrus Raspberry Chia Seed Pudding (p 263)	1 slice Yacon Roasted Pineapple (p 287)	3 Dark Chocolate–Covered Pichuberries (p 265)	1 slice Yacon Roasted Pineapple (p 287)	1 Yummy Stuffed Date with Cacao and Walnuts (p 288)	1 Dark Chocolate Fig with Cacao Nibs (p 267)

VEGETARIAN 1800 CALORIE 7-DAY MENU

	MONDAY	TUESDAY	WEDNESDAY	THURSDAY	FRIDAY	SATURDAY	SUNDAY
BREAKFAST	½ cup Oven-Roasted Pichuberries (p 217), 8 egg whites (1 cup), scrambled, 1 slice whole grain bread, toasted	1½ cups Sweet Potato Crustless Quiche (p 87), 1 cup cubed papaya	2 tablespoons Pichuberry Marmalade (p 247), 2 slices whole grain bread, toasted, 4 ounces skim queso fresco cheese	2 cups Power-Packed Incan Parfait (p 75)	1 Quinoa Pichuberry Muffin (p 83), 6 egg whites (¾ cup), scrambled, 1 cup salsa	Make a shake: 1 cup unsweetened almond milk, 1 cup berries, vegetarian protein powder (20–25g protein), 1 tablespoon chia seeds	2 slices Overnight Lucuma French Toast (p 71), 1 tablespoon yacon syrup (or 2 teaspoons agave), 1 hardboiled egg
SNACK	¼ cup Avocado Hummus (p 241), 1 cup vegetable sticks	Make a shake: 1 cup unsweetened almond milk, ¾ cup berries, vegetarian protein powder (20–25g protein)	¼ cup Power Trail Mix (p 221)	1 Inca Power Bar (p 215)	¾ cup berries, ¾ cup low-fat Greek yogurt	½ cup unsweetened applesauce, 1 tablespoon chia seeds	¼ cup Roasted Garlic Artichoke Dip (p 251), 1 cup vegetable sticks
LUNCH	1 White Bean Avocado Wrap (p 187), 3½ cups mixed greens, 2 tablespoons lemon juice, 1 cup Chicha Tisane (p 37)	2 cups Garbanzo Saltado (p 109), 6 cups raw spinach, steamed, 1 tablespoon lemon juice, 1 cup Chicha Tisane (p 37)	3 skewers Tofu à la Panca (p 145), ½ cup black beans, 3½ cups mixed greens, 2 tablespoons lemon juice, 1 cup Chicha Tisane (p 37)	3 cups Minestrone with Quinoa Noodles (p 197), 3½ cups mixed greens, 2 tablespoons lemon juice, 1 cup Chicha Tisane (p 37)	3 Black Bean & Sweet Potato Thai Fusion Tacos (p 165), 1 cup Chicha Tisane (p 37)	2½ cups Butternut Squash & Legumes Quinoa Salad (p 167), 5 tablespoons Cucumber-Cilantro Lime Dressing (p 245), 1 cup Chicha Tisane (p 37)	1½ cups Zesty Vegan Chickpea Salad (p 190), 1 whole grain pita bread, 1 cup lettuce, ¼ tomato, 1 cup Chicha Tisane (p 37)
SNACK	½ Boiled Sweet Potato (p 234), ¾ cup low-fat Greek yogurt, 4 walnut halves	½ cup unsweetened applesauce, 1 tablespoon chia seeds	1 medium apple, 1 hard-boiled egg	¼ cup Roasted Garlic Artichoke Dip (p 251), 1 ounce crackers	1 Inca Power Bar (p 215)	¼ cup Avocado Hummus (p 241), 1 cup vegetable sticks	¼ cup Power Trail Mix (p 221)
DINNER	2 cups Arroz con Tofu (p 101), ½ cup Salsa Criolla (p 253)	3 slices Tempeh Milanese (p 143), ½ cup cooked pasta, ½ cup marinara sauce	1 cup Trigo Guisado (p 209), 1 cup cooked broccoli, 2 tablespoons lemon juice	2 cups Garlic Butter Beans à la Parmesan (p 110), 1 (3 ounce) vegetarian sausage, 3½ cups mixed greens, 2 tablespoons lemon juice, 1 cup Chicha Tisane (p 37)	2 cups Tofu Vegetable Aji Panca Curry (p 207), 1 cup black rice	1½ cups Aji de Tempeh (p 98), 1 cup cooked zucchini, 1 hard-boiled egg	1 cup Artichoke Seitan Molido (p 103), ½ cup brown rice, 2 tablespoons avocado
TREAT	5 Dark Chocolate-Covered Pichuberries (p 265)	1 cup Citrus Raspberry Chia Seed Pudding (p 263)	1 slice Yacon Roasted Pineapple (p 287)	5 Dark Chocolate-Covered Pichuberries (p 265)	1 slice Yacon Roasted Pineapple (p 287)	1 Yummy Stuffed Date with Cacao and Walnuts (p 288)	1 Dark Chocolate Fig with Cacao Nibs (p 267)

For optimal weight loss, where you lose fat and maintain lean muscle mass, your weight loss efforts should be 80 percent nutrition and 20 percent exercise. This is the 80/20 Rule. I am a fierce advocate for exercising for health. *However, exercise is not the primary means to lose weight. It's not about how much you exercise to lose weight. It's about how much you eat to lose weight.* Be as active as you can be, but remember that what you put in your mouth is what will speed up or inhibit your weight loss. Here are the guidelines for exercise.

Low-Intensity Reboot Exercise

Examples: walking, hatha yoga, stretching, easy swimming, light weight training, bicycling less than 5 mph, golfing using a cart, light yard work or housework.

Needs: All the meal plans provide you with two daily snacks. Make sure to have a snack before the workout. This is all you need for fuel, regardless of how many times a week you work out at a low intensity.

High-Intensity Reboot Exercise

Examples: circuit training, CrossFit, boot camps, high-intensity body-pumping classes, spinning, running for forty-five minutes or more, boxing, kickboxing, intense swimming, vigorous dance classes.

Needs: People who exercise at a high intensity should include the extra pre-workout maca reboot shake (the shake is not shown in the sample meal plans). If you are working out, drink the shake forty-five minutes to one hour prior to the activity. Stay fueled and do not create a bigger deficit between energy expended and energy consumed. Losing fat is not about deprivation and eating little amounts of food. You want to stay powered and energized so you can blast the belly fat, reboot your body, and get that waistline you've always wanted.

Maca Reboot Pre-Exercise Shake

Stories tell us that the Incans would take maca before fighting in the wars for optimal strength and vitality, increased energy, and decreased chronic fatigue. Nowadays, South American soccer players take maca before game time to enhance strength and performance. Maca is a root vegetable, comparable to turnips or radishes, that is found in the Andes of Peru and is packed full of calcium, iron, magnesium, and all essential amino acids that prevent muscle breakdown, keep bones strong, and minimize fatigue. Research shows that the amino acid profile and mineral content of maca assists with boosting energy. Maca also has vitamin C and various B vitamins necessary for our body's functionality, and it's amazing for optimal sports nutrition. To feel the effects of maca, you need to consume the shake four to five times per week, not just once a week or on a sporadic basis. Enjoy the shake forty-five minutes to one hour before the workout.

Maca has a positive effect on energy and mood, making it a perfect pre-workout supplement. It can even support continued exercise after extended effort because studies show it increases glucose in the bloodstream after a prolonged fast. Research also suggests that maca boosts energy because of its amino acid profile and mineral content.

Warmi (Female) Power Pre-Exercise Shake	Qhari (Male) Power Pre-Exercise Shake
2 teaspoons maca	1 tablespoon maca
1 medium banana, 5 to 6 inches	1 medium banana, 7 to 8 inches
1 tablespoon cacao powder	1 tablespoon cacao powder
1 cup of milk of choice (cow, rice, almond, or soy)	1 cup of milk of choice (cow, rice, almond, or soy)
15–20g of protein powder of choice (whey, rice, pea, or soy)	20–25g of protein powder of choice (whey, rice, pea, or soy)

DIRECTIONS:

❶ Put all the ingredients in a blender and puree until the shake is the desired consistency.

Sweets

Cacao helps with appetite regulation and weight loss. Raw cacao is rich in antioxidants, essential minerals, vitamins, and natural mood-enhancing nutrients called theobromine and phenylethylamine. The latter is a super low-potency antidepressant that works like the body's dopamine and adrenaline. Cacao can increase the amount of serotonin your brain produces, which can create a balancing effect and sense of well-being. In addition, cacao is a natural appetite suppressant, so it can help reduce food cravings and aid in weight loss. Numerous studies show that cacao phenolics lower insulin resistance and sensitivity, so it may be useful in managing diabetes, too. Many of our recipes have cacao in them, so you will be satisfied, nourished, and full.

Remember: treats are treats and need to be regulated and portion-controlled. There's nothing wrong with wanting to finish a meal with a sweet delicacy. Fighting your sweet tooth can cause problems of bingeing or overconsumption. We've incorporated many pleasurable indulgences in all the various meal plans. Make the recipes. Enjoy the right portion for you and experience the love as needed.

Dining Out

We understand you cannot stop your life while losing weight. You will continue to socialize, go out with friends and family, and enjoy your time with others.

Top Tips When Dining Out

♦ Dine out no more than one to two times per week for optimal success.

♦ Savor the meal and enjoy it instead of worrying or feeling guilty. By dining out only one to two times per week and following the meal plans we have provided for you, you will succeed in losing weight. Enjoy the minimal splurges.

♦ Planning ahead makes all the difference. If possible, go online to see the choices available and pick a dish that works for your goals.

♦ If you must eat out more than once or twice a week, you need to be more cautious. Have a snack before going to the restaurant so you are not starving when you get there. You will make better food choices and be less enticed to eat the bread or chips on the table.

♦ Start with a salad or soup. What you'll discover is, after an appetizer, you may feel fuller. Choose an appetizer as your entrée or cut your entrée in half and eat less of it.

♦ Ask for sauces and dressings on the side. This may sound obvious, but you wouldn't believe how many people order these extras on the side and then proceed to pour them all over their meal, using every last drop. It kind of defeats the purpose of getting it on the side in the first place, right? The whole point is that you should use about half the amount of what most restaurants provide. Waiters may tell you things are lightly dressed, but that is rarely the case.

♦ *Remember:* it's useful to think of eating out as celebratory. I treat it as ordering something exotic and rewarding that I only allow myself once in a while.

Drinking alcohol is definitely a choice that only you alone can make. Moderation is important, so if you do drink alcohol, it can be worked into your plan. Take note that, when your liver is processing alcohol, it cannot process fat—it only does one function at a time. So, the fact that you're not metabolizing fat when you're drinking means you're holding on to fats that would otherwise be processed.

Tips for Alcohol Consumption

◆ Think of a drink as a special occasion situation and not a daily habit.

◆ Consume no more than four to six servings of alcohol per week for ideal weight loss.

◆ For weight loss, there's no specific research, but what I've observed is that men may have six servings per week, while women may have four servings per week.

◆ *Serving sizes:* 1 serving of alcohol is equivalent to 4 ounces of wine, a shot of booze (1.5 ounces), or 12 ounces of beer.

◆ The oversized globe wineglasses in restaurants contain 6 ounces a pour (one and a half servings). A glass of wine in your house usually equals 8 ounces (two servings). Cocktails in restaurants may include two shots and equal two servings.

◆ Alcohol stimulates appetite, which puts you at risk for higher calorie intake. Alcohol also lowers your inhibitions, making it easier to choose unhealthy foods.

◆ Many people enjoy a glass of wine with dinner as a matter of course, or because they are foodies. Instead of wine at every dinner, enjoy it when you're at restaurants, on weekends, or once a week, not every day. Remember that, when you are drinking alcohol, your body is not metabolizing fat, which is counter to your weight loss efforts.

Long-Term Success & Maintenance

Congratulations! You've made it to the final phase of the Whole Body Reboot plan, which is to maintain your weight loss goals throughout your daily life. This phase emphasizes the positive patterns and habits you need to develop to maintain lifelong success with your health and wellness. By following these guidelines, you'll experience amazing antiaging benefits. You will be full of energy, vitality, and internal strength. Your body will appreciate all the superfoods you consume on a daily basis, and you'll feel like an Incan warrior.

Warmi (Female) Plan

For women, you will increase your overall food intake by 25 percent of your original 1,300-calorie weight loss plan. What this means is that throughout the day, you will be adding in additional food at your meals and snacks in order to maintain the weight you have achieved.

For example:

- **Add a piece of fruit at breakfast or as a snack (one more fruit per day).**
- **Add 2 ounces of protein at lunch and dinner (4 ounces per day).**
- **Add ¼ cup of extra grain or starch at lunch and dinner (½ cup total per day).**

- Continue to consume your maca reboot pre-exercise shake (keep as active as you can to help maintain your success).

By adding in these extra food sources, you will increase your intake by 25 percent and maintain your long-term success. Continue to follow the menus and incorporate the other mouthwatering recipes in the book to enjoy a life of variety, diversity, superfoods, and flavor.

Quari (Male) Plan

For men, you will increase your overall food intake by 35 percent of your original 1,800-calorie weight loss plan. What this means is that throughout the day, you will be adding in additional food at your meals and snacks in order to maintain the weight you have achieved. For example:

- Add ½ cup extra grain and starch at breakfast.
- Add a piece of fruit at breakfast and as a snack (two more fruits per day).
- Add 3 ounces of protein at lunch and dinner (6 ounces per day).
- Add ½ cup of extra grain and starch at lunch and dinner (1 cup total per day).
- Continue to consume your maca reboot pre-exercise shake (keep as active as you can to help maintain your success).

You have now increased your daily food intake by 35 percent to maintain lifelong success. Enjoy the menus, check out the additional recipes in the book, and continue to live an antiaging life of super health and wellness.

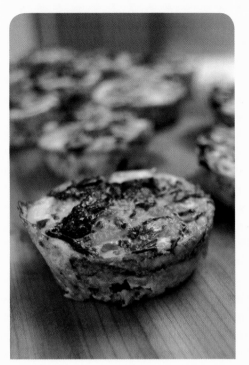
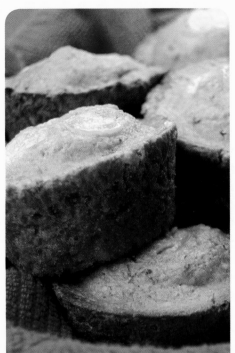

CHAPTER 4

Breakfast

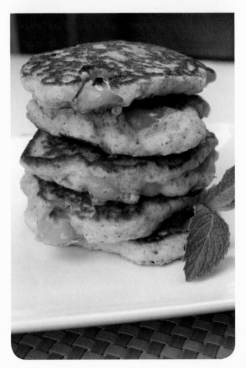

BREAKFAST BRAIN-FOOD PARFAIT

Servings: 1 ♦ Serving size: 1¾ cups

¾ cup low-fat Greek yogurt

¾ cup mixed berries

1 tablespoon crushed walnuts

1 tablespoon cacao nibs

1 tablespoon chia seeds

1 tablespoon honey *or* agave

Experience a super combination of omega-3 health from multiple sources. Start your day off right with this parfait, and power your brain toward optimal function.

1 Put the yogurt in a serving bowl. Top with the berries, walnuts, nibs, seeds, and honey or agave. Eat immediately or take it on the go.

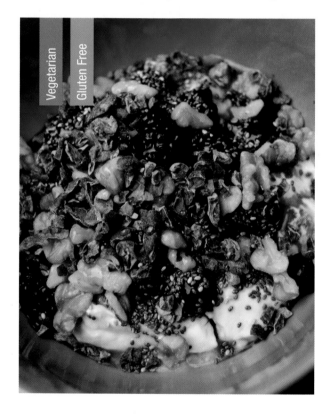

Chia seeds have recently gained attention as an excellent source of omega-3 fatty acid. They are also an excellent source of fiber at 10 grams per ounce (about 2 tablespoons) and contain protein and minerals, including iron, calcium, magnesium, and zinc.

Per Serving: Kcal 407, Protein 22.5g, Carb 46.5g, Fat 17.5g, Sodium 73mg, Dietary Fiber 11g
Daily Values: Fiber 44%, Vit C 7%, Vit A 4%, Vit D 5 0%, Calcium 30%, Iron 17%

BREAKFAST OF CHAMPIONS
À LA PERUVIAN

Servings: 1 ♦ Serving size: About 2 cups

This is not your typical boxed cereal. It will rock your health and wellness using superfoods galore.

1 Put the popped kiwicha in a bowl. Top with the pichuberries, chia seeds, cacao nibs, and walnuts. Serve with milk of choice.

½ cup popped kiwicha
(see recipe on page 220)

½ cup pichuberries, halved

1 tablespoon chia seeds

1 tablespoon cacao nibs

1 tablespoon chopped walnuts

1 cup of milk of choice

Vegan

Gluten Free

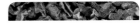

Cacao is rich in essential vitamins A, B1, B2, B3, C, E, and pantothenic acid. It also contains a high amount of polyphenols. In addition, cacao beans are loaded with essential minerals like calcium, copper, iron, magnesium, manganese, potassium, and zinc.

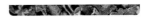

Per Serving: Kcal 343, Protein 16g, Carb 42g, Fat 15g, Sodium 147mg, Dietary Fiber 9g
Daily Values: Fiber 35%, Vit C 16%, Vit A 34%, Vit D 5 58%, Calcium 40%, Iron 16%

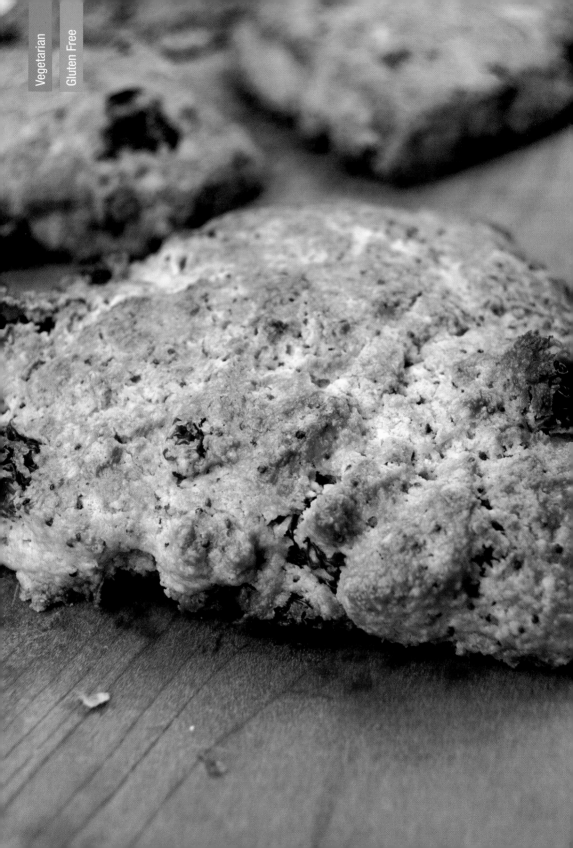

GLUTEN-FREE PICHUBERRY SCONE

Servings: 8 ♦ Serving size: 1 wedge

Enjoy this wholesome pichuberry scone for a healthful, sweet morning treat. We thank Chenoa Bol, our friend and pastry chef, for providing us with this mouthwatering recipe. I originally challenged her to make a low-fat scone, and she stated, "Manuel, it's a scone." We laughed, and she developed this delicious gluten-free recipe.

½ cup unsalted butter, cold

2 cups oat flour

⅓ cup packed light brown sugar

1 teaspoon baking powder

¼ teaspoon baking soda

½ teaspoon salt

½ cup dried pichuberries (or dried blueberries or cranberries)

½ cup low-fat Greek yogurt

1 egg

❶ Preheat the oven to 400 degrees F. Line a cookie sheet with parchment paper.

❷ Using a cheese grater, grate the butter onto a large plate and place it in the freezer to harden.

❸ In a medium bowl, combine the flour, sugar, baking powder, baking soda, and salt. Add the frozen butter, working it into the flour mixture until it resembles coarse meal. Add the dried pichuberries and mix to combine.

❹ In a small bowl, whisk the yogurt and egg to combine. Add the wet mixture to the dry mixture and gently stir with a rubber spatula until the dough comes together.

❺ Put the dough on a lightly floured surface. Flatten it into an 8- to 9-inch round. Cut the round into eight wedges. Gently transfer the wedges to the cookie sheet, placing them 2 inches apart from one another.

❻ Bake until golden, for 20 to 25 minutes. Serve warm or at room temperature.

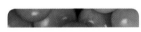

Pichuberries have a high content of phenolic compounds (phenols), which are natural antioxidants. Vitamin C and phenolic compounds are known to be great free radical scavengers. Free radicals cause oxidation, which can lead to many chronic diseases.

Per Serving: Kcal 269, Protein 6g, Carb 30g, Fat 15g, Sodium 259.5mg, Dietary Fiber 3g
Daily Values: Fiber 12%, Vit C 1%, Vit A 20%, Vit D 5 3%, Calcium 5%, Iron 2%

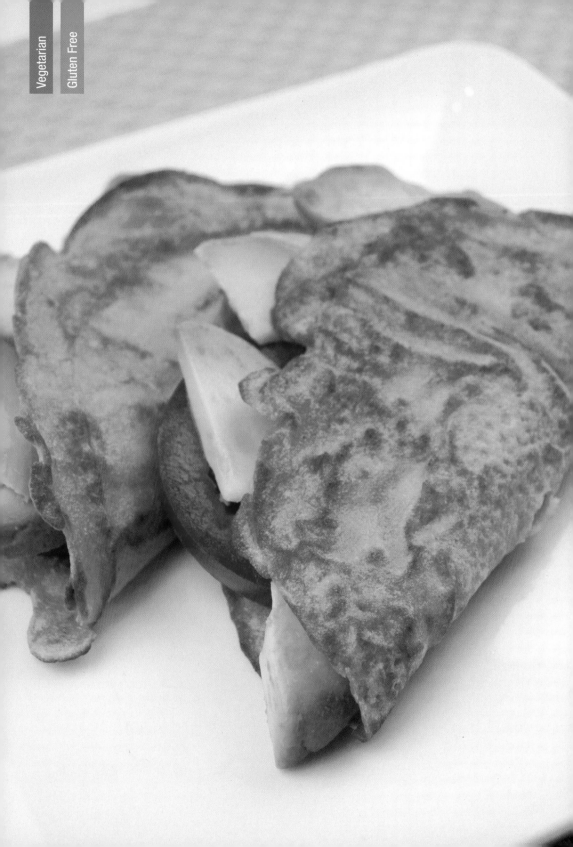

GLUTEN-FREE QUINOA CREPE

Servings: 7 ♦ Serving Size: One 8-inch crepe

The French love their crepes, and we wanted you to experience the classic French recipe specially modified for your gluten-free needs. You can fill your crepe with anything your heart desires. Try tomatoes, avocados, or even Nutella. Bon appétit!

1 egg

¼ cup low-fat milk

¼ cup water

½ cup quinoa flour

Pinch of salt

1 tablespoon canola oil

Oil spray

❶ Put the egg, milk, water, flour, and salt in a blender and pulse until combined. Scrape down the edges of the blender.

❷ Add the canola oil to the blender and pulse to combine.

❸ Heat an 8-inch nonstick sauté pan over medium-low heat. Spray with an even coat of oil. When the pan is hot, lift it from the heat and pour about 3 tablespoons of batter into the corner of the pan. Immediately swirl the batter to coat the bottom of the pan, then place the pan back on the heat for about a minute or until the crepe is set.

❹ Using a rubber spatula to loosen it from the surface of the pan, flip the crepe. Cook the other side for 30 seconds and then remove.

❺ Repeat the process with the remaining batter, making sure to oil the pan for each crepe.

Quinoa is rich in B vitamins, calcium, copper, iron, magnesium, vitamins C and E, and zinc.

Per Serving: Kcal 49.5, Protein 2g, Carb 3g, Fat 3g, Sodium 98mg, Dietary Fiber 1g
Daily Values: Fiber 1%, Vit C 0%, Vit A 1%, Vit D 5 2%, Calcium 2%, Iron 2%

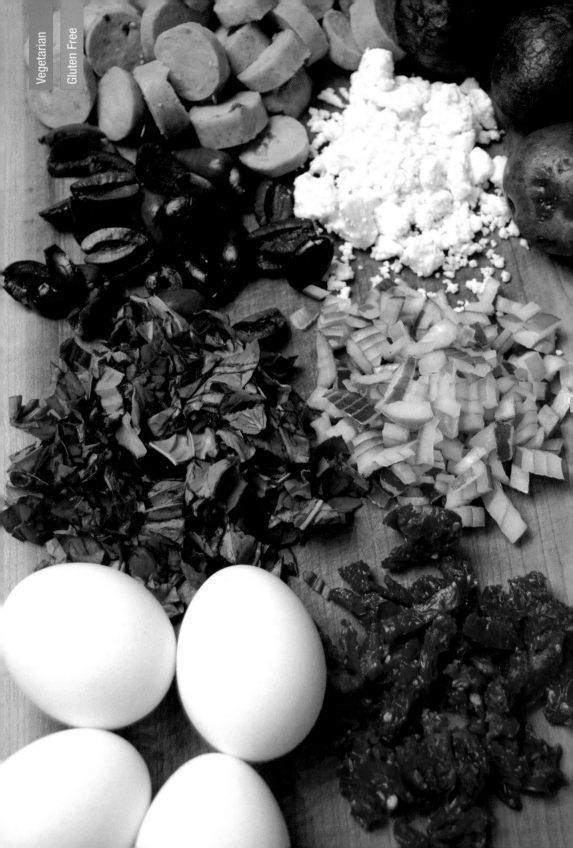

MEDITERRANEAN PERUVIAN FUSION SCRAMBLE

Servings: 4 ♦ Serving size: 1½ cups

This will transport you to the Mediterranean Sea overlooking the water while tasting classic flavors, including olives, tomatoes, and cheese. We've infused the Mediterranean with a Peruvian flare by using purple potatoes. Let the adventure begin!

❶ Preheat the oven to 400 degrees F. Lightly spray a sheet pan with oil.

❷ Place the potato rounds on the sheet pan and season with salt and pepper to taste. Bake until tender, for 30 to 40 minutes.

❸ While the potatoes are baking, make the scramble. Heat the oil in a large sauté pan over medium heat. When the oil is hot, add the onion and sauté until softened, for about 5 minutes.

❹ Add the sausage, tomatoes, and olives. Sauté until the sausage is cooked through. Turn off the heat and toss with the feta cheese and basil. Serve warm over the roasted potatoes.

Oil spray

4 small purple potatoes, cut into ½-inch thick rounds

Salt and pepper

1 tablespoon olive oil

⅓ cup chopped red onion

2 chicken sausages, sliced

¼ cup sliced sundried tomatoes, rehydrated

¼ cup sliced Kalamata olives

¼ cup crumbled feta cheese

⅓ cup chopped basil

Purple potatoes pack two to three times the antioxidants of yellow or white potatoes, which means more free radical scavenging. They are also rich in anthocyanins, the phytochemicals responsible for their purple color and their impressive health benefits.

Per Serving: Kcal 337, Protein 16g, Carb 45g, Fat 10g, Sodium 1263mg, Dietary Fiber 3.5g
Daily Values: Fiber 14%, Vit C 7%, Vit A 7%, Vit D 5 0%, Calcium 7%, Iron 7%

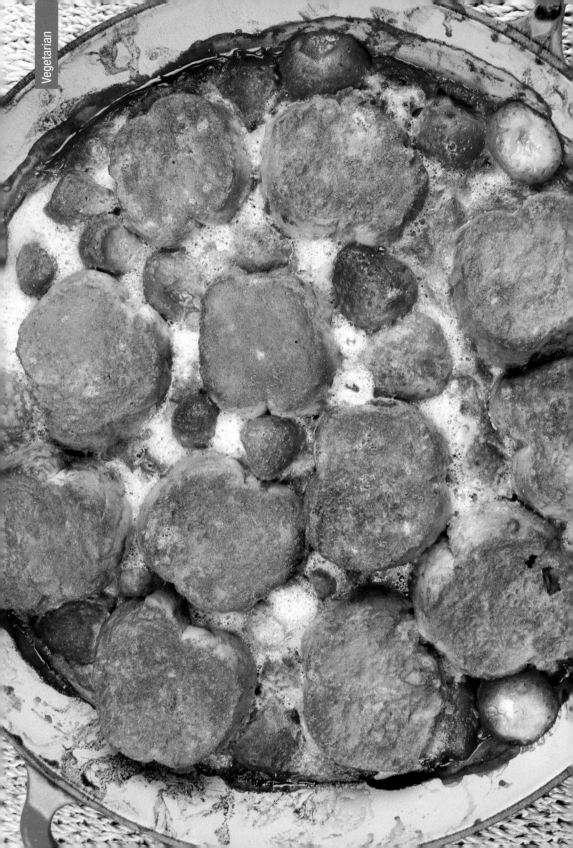

OVERNIGHT LUCUMA FRENCH TOAST

Servings: 12 ♦ Serving size: One 1½-inch slice

Make the French toast the night before so that in the morning you can just pop it in the oven for a warm, sweet breakfast—delightful for the entire family.

1 French baguette *(18 inches long)*, sliced into 1½-inch-thick slices

5 large eggs

¾ cup low-fat milk

1 tablespoon vanilla extract

¾ cup lucuma powder

½ teaspoon ground cinnamon

¼ teaspoon baking powder

1 package *(16 ounces)* **frozen whole strawberries, thawed**

Oil spray

❶ Place the bread slices in a casserole dish large enough to fit the slices in a single layer without leaving too much unoccupied space.

❷ Combine the eggs, milk, vanilla, lucuma, cinnamon, and baking powder in a medium-size bowl and whisk to combine. Pour the egg mixture over the bread slices. Cover with plastic wrap and refrigerate for 8 hours or overnight. Flip the slices over about halfway through the soaking process (or just before baking if left to soak overnight).

❸ Preheat the oven to 450 degrees F. Lightly oil a baking dish that is slightly larger than the dish used for soaking.

❹ Transfer the bread slices to the baking dish and pour any remaining egg mixture over the bread. Fill in the gaps between the bread slices with thawed whole strawberries.

❺ Bake for 15 minutes or until golden and set.

Lucuma is a natural sweetener with a very low glycemic index of 25, which makes it a safe alternative for diabetics and great for weight loss.

Per Serving: Kcal 296, Protein 9.5g, Carb 41g, Fat 3g, Sodium 350.5mg, Dietary Fiber 2g
Daily Values: Fiber 7%, Vit C 37%, Vit A 3%, Vit D 5 4%, Calcium 6%, Iron 14%

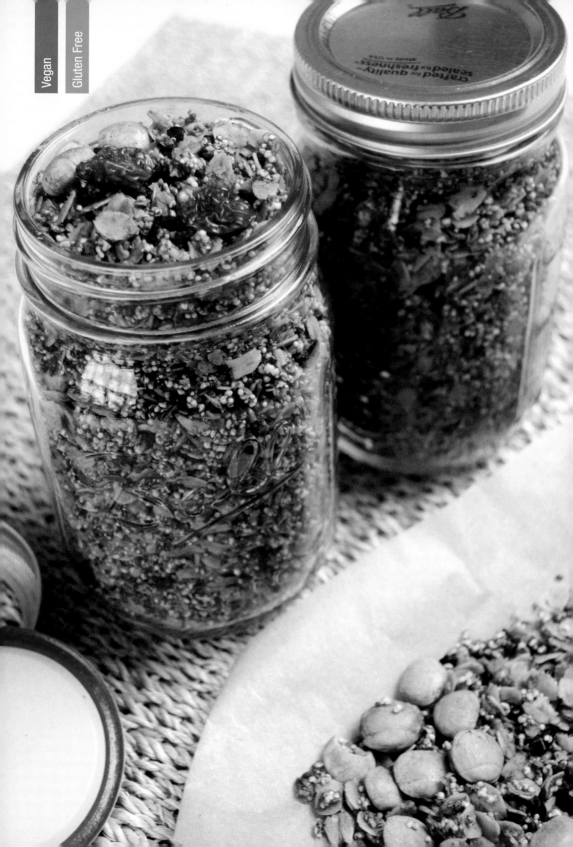

PERUVIAN KIWICHA GRANOLA

Servings: 12 ◆ Serving size: ½ cup

Experience a crunch of power with every bite of this super simple-to-make granola.

① Preheat the oven to 300 degrees F.

② In a large bowl, combine the popped kiwicha, oats, coconut, sacha inchi seeds, pichuberries, cacao nibs, and cinnamon. Using a wooden spoon, toss to combine.

③ Put the coconut oil and agave syrup in a small saucepan over low heat. When melted, pour over the granola mixture and toss to thoroughly coat.

④ Evenly distribute the granola mixture over a parchment-lined sheet pan. Bake for 30 to 40 minutes, stirring every 10 minutes, until the granola is fragrant and golden.

⑤ Transfer the cooled granola to jars and store at room temperature for one to two weeks.

2 cups popped kiwicha *(see recipe on page 220)*

2 cups old-fashioned rolled oats

½ cup shredded unsweetened coconut

½ cup sacha inchi seeds *(or almonds)*

½ cup dried pichuberries *(or dried blueberries)*

½ cup cacao nibs

1 tablespoon ground cinnamon

3 tablespoons coconut oil

5 tablespoons agave syrup

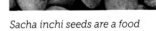

Sacha inchi seeds are a food that's naturally, perfectly balanced, offering the optimum ratio of omega-3 and omega-6 fatty acids. That's important because the balance between these two types of fatty acids has been proven to decrease risk factors for chronic diseases.

Per Serving: Kcal 217, Protein 5g, Carb 28.5g, Fat 10g, Sodium 6.5mg, Dietary Fiber 14g
Daily Values: Fiber 14%, Vit C 1%, Vit A 8%, Vit D 5 0%, Calcium 2%, Iron 8%

POWER MORNING SPINACH EGG-WHITE OMELET

Servings: 1 ◆ Serving size: 1 omelet

This is a basic, easy-to-make, low-fat, classic omelet. Make it in 5 minutes for a light breakfast.

2 teaspoons olive oil

2 cups spinach

Salt and pepper

½ cup liquid egg whites

DIRECTIONS:

❶ Heat 1 teaspoon of the oil in a small sauté pan over medium heat. When the oil is hot, add the spinach and salt and pepper to taste. Cook the spinach until wilted, then transfer it to a small bowl and set aside.

❷ Using the same sauté pan, heat the remaining oil over medium heat. Add the egg whites and salt and pepper to taste. Cook the omelet until firm on one side. Using a rubber spatula, carefully flip the omelet to cook the other side.

❸ When the egg is cooked throughout, gently slide the omelet onto a plate and fill with the cooked spinach. Serve immediately.

Per Serving: Kcal 112.5, Protein 15g, Carb 3g, Fat 5g, Sodium 249.5mg, Dietary Fiber 1.5g
Daily Values: Fiber 6%, Vit C 28%, Vit A 0%, Vit D 5 0%, Calcium 7%, Iron 10%

POWER-PACKED INCAN PARFAIT

Servings: 1 ◆ Serving size: Approximately 2 cups

This is a perfect recipe to make ahead so you have a few days' worth of grab-'n'-go breakfast options. Put the power-packed Incan parfait in a mason jar for easy travel and convenience.

1 cup cubed papaya

¾ cup low-fat Greek yogurt

¾ cup popped kiwicha *(see recipe on page 220)*

2 tablespoons walnut pieces

1 Put ½ cup of the papaya in a wide-mouthed mason jar, followed by 3 tablespoons of the yogurt and 3 tablespoons of the popped kiwicha. Layer the remaining papaya, yogurt, and kiwicha in the jar and top with the walnuts. Eat as is or put a cover on it and store it in the refrigerator for tomorrow's breakfast.

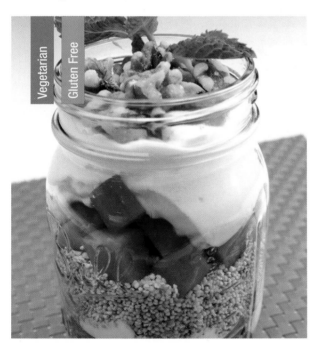

Vegetarian Gluten Free

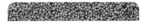

Kiwicha is rich in iron, magnesium, manganese, phosphorus, and soluble and insoluble fiber; it's also low in sodium. Loaded with phytochemicals like squalene, it also is a great source of natural antioxidants. Squalene has been shown to promote positive changes in the immune system and to prevent cancer.

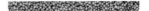

Per Serving: Kcal 383, Protein 24g, Carb 41g, Fat 15g, Sodium 80mg, Dietary Fiber 6g
Daily Values: Fiber 24%, Vit C 146%, Vit A 31%, Vit D 5 0%, Calcium 29%, Iron 15%

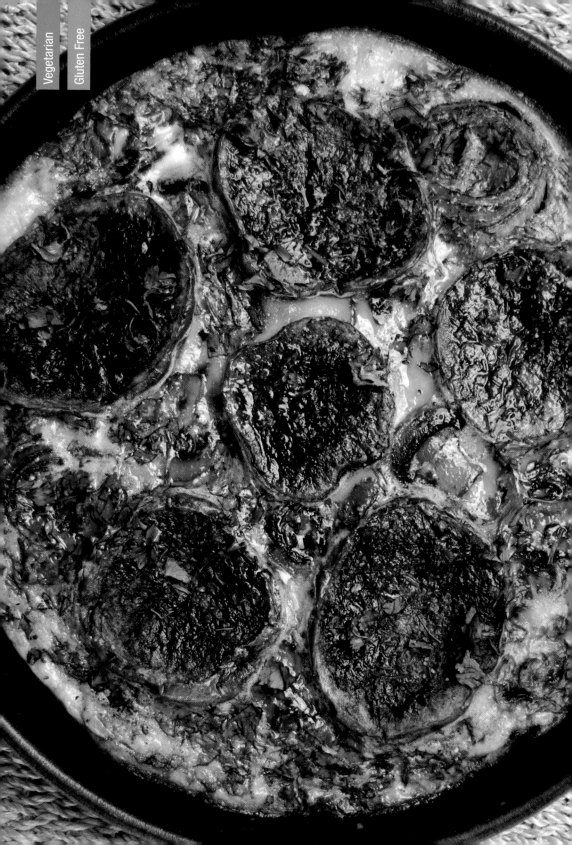

PURPLE POTATO FRITTATA

Servings: 6 ◆ Serving size: 1 wedge

This traditional Italian-inspired frittata is infused with Peruvian power foods to enhance your breakfast and optimize your energy.

Oil spray

3 medium purple potatoes, cut into ½-inch-thick rounds

½ medium yellow onion, sliced into ½-inch-thick rounds

Salt and pepper

3 cups sliced mushrooms

2 cups spinach

6 eggs

2 tablespoons ají amarillo paste (or mild chili paste)

¼ cup chopped cilantro

❶ Preheat the oven to 400 degrees F. Lightly spray a sheet pan with oil.

❷ Place the potato and onion slices on the pan. Season with salt and pepper to taste. Bake vegetables until tender, for 30 to 40 minutes.

❸ While the potatoes and onions are roasting, lightly spray a medium sauté pan with oil and place it over medium heat. When the pan is hot, add the mushrooms and the spinach. Cook until the vegetables are lightly wilted. Season with salt and pepper and set aside.

❹ Put the eggs, ají, and cilantro in a small bowl and whisk to combine. Set aside.

❺ When the potatoes and onions are done, remove them from the oven (leaving the oven on) and arrange half of them in the bottom of a well-oiled 8-inch cast-iron pan. Top with the spinach mixture and the remaining potatoes and onions.

❻ Place the cast-iron pan over medium heat. When you hear crackling, pour the egg mixture over the top. Continue cooking the frittata on the stove top until the sides set and become slightly puffy, for 5 to 7 minutes.

❼ Immediately transfer the frittata to the preheated oven to bake the top, for 5 to 7 minutes longer. Frittata should be slightly puffy and golden on top. Let the frittata cool slightly before serving.

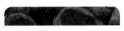

When you eat purple potatoes, the anthocyanins are absorbed directly into the bloodstream, which has a healing effect on the liver and helps to decrease blood pressure.

Per Serving: Kcal 168, Protein 7g, Carb 24g, Fat 5g, Sodium 120mg, Dietary Fiber 2.5g
Daily Values: Fiber 2.5%, Vit C 10%, Vit A 6%, Vit D 5 7%, Calcium 4%, Iron 6%

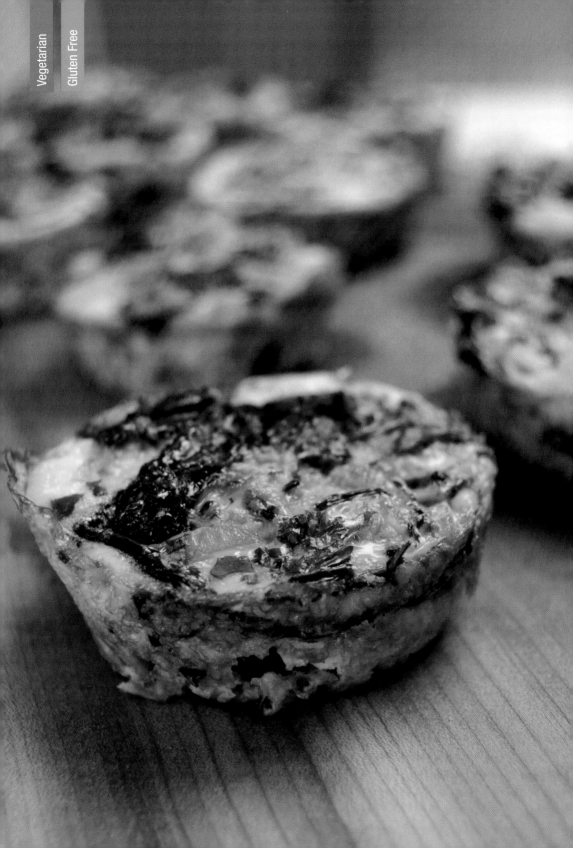

QUINOA, SPINACH & EGG-WHITE MUFFINS

Servings: 12 ◆ Serving size: 1 muffin

Looking for a quick breakfast? Bake these muffins in advance and fuel yourself throughout the week.

1 Heat the oil in a medium-size sauté pan over medium heat. When the oil is hot, add the onions and garlic. Sauté for a few minutes until the onions become transparent. Add the spinach and salt and pepper to taste. Cook just until the spinach wilts. Remove from the heat and let cool completely before proceeding to the next step.

2 Preheat the oven to 350 degrees F.

3 Transfer the cooled spinach mixture to a medium-size mixing bowl, along with the cilantro, quinoa, and egg whites. Mix to combine.

4 Lightly spray a muffin tin with oil. Put ¼ cup of the muffin batter into each of the muffin cups. Top off with any remaining batter.

5 Bake for 10 to 15 minutes until lightly golden and puffy. Let the muffins cool slightly before removing them from the tin.

* If using whole eggs instead of liquid egg whites, it will take approximately 16 whole eggs to yield 2 cups of egg whites.

1 tablespoon olive oil

½ medium yellow onion, diced

2 cloves garlic, crushed

6 cups spinach

Salt and pepper

½ cup chopped cilantro

1 cup cooked quinoa *(see recipe on page 238)*

2 cups liquid egg whites *(such as All Whites 100% Liquid Egg Whites)**

Oil spray

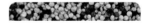

Quinoa contains a total of twenty-one amino acids. Eleven of these can be synthesized by our bodies and are therefore nonessential. However, the ten remaining essential amino acids make quinoa a complete protein.

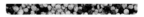

Per Serving: Kcal 50.5, Protein 5g, Carb 4g, Fat 1.5g, Sodium 73mg, Dietary Fiber 1.5g
Daily Values: Fiber 5%, Vit C 8%, Vit A 1%, Vit D 5 0%, Calcium 2%, Iron 4%

QUINOA CRANBERRY COCO FUSION

Servings: 6 ♦ Serving size: 1²/₃ cups

3 cups cooked quinoa
(see recipe on page 238)

16 ounces *(1 block)* light silken tofu, cut into small cubes

½ cup dried cranberries

½ cup shredded unsweetened coconut

4 cups unsweetened almond milk

1 teaspoon ground cinnamon

A pleasingly warm breakfast you can make the night before and reheat in the morning.

❶ Put all of the ingredients in a medium saucepan over medium-low heat. Cook, stirring frequently, until heated throughout. Serve warm.

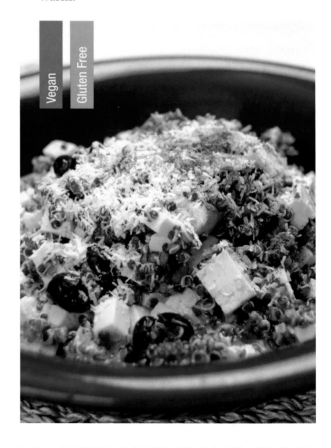

Vegan Gluten Free

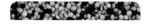

Quinoa contains essential fatty acids (EFAs), specifically linoleic acid and linolenic acid. Consuming these polyunsaturated fatty acids has been linked to improved blood sugar control and cardiovascular health.

Per Serving: Kcal 166, Protein 5g, Carb 23.5g, Fat 6g, Sodium 136mg, Dietary Fiber 2.5g
Daily Values: Fiber 10%, Vit C 1%, Vit A 7%, Vit D 5 17%, Calcium 4%, Iron 14%

QUINOA PUMPKIN PORRIDGE

Servings: 4 ◆ Serving size: 1 cup

Experience a sweet porridge without all the sugar while enjoying powerful spices, carotenoids, and one of our favorite superfoods: quinoa.

❶ Put all the ingredients in a large saucepan and stir to combine. Bring to a boil over medium heat, then lower to a simmer. Cover the pan and cook for 15 to 20 minutes or until the quinoa is fluffy and completely cooked.

NOTE: Serve this warm with a sprinkling of walnuts and shredded coconut or other healthful toppings of your choice.

1 cup quinoa

1 can *(15 ounces)* pumpkin puree

1 cup water

1 cup low-fat milk

¼ cup agave syrup

1 teaspoon ground cinnamon

½ teaspoon ground ginger

½ teaspoon ground nutmeg

¼ teaspoon ground cloves

¼ teaspoon ground allspice

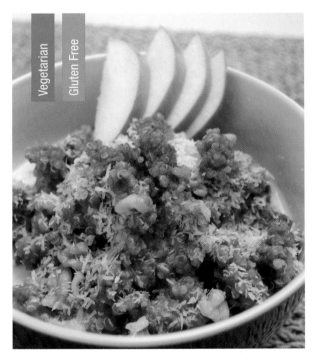

Vegetarian | Gluten Free

Seasoning a high-carb food with cinnamon can help prevent a spike in your blood sugar levels. Cinnamon slows the rate of gastric emptying after meals, steadying the rise in blood sugar levels after eating.

Per Serving: Kcal 309, Protein 10.5g, Carb 57.5g, Fat 4.5g, Sodium 44.5mg, Dietary Fiber 14.5g
Daily Values: Fiber 58%, Vit C 8%, Vit A 337%, Vit D 5 8%, Calcium 13%, Iron 24%

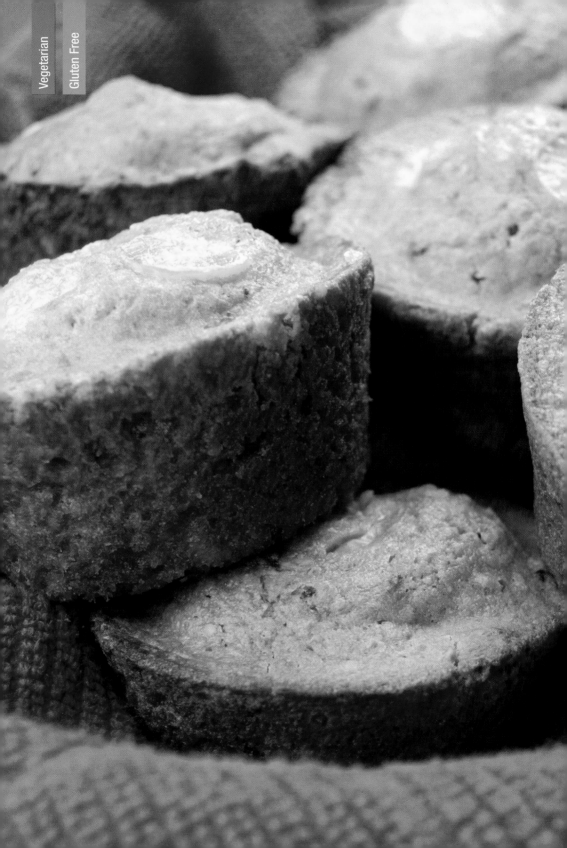

QUINOA PICHUBERRY MUFFINS

Servings: 12 ◆ Serving size: 1 muffin

Looking for a nutritious baked delight? You've found your match! Enjoy these muffins for breakfast or a snack.

Oil spray

2 cups oat flour

1 teaspoon salt

1 teaspoon baking powder

1 teaspoon baking soda

2 cups pichuberries

¼ cup low-fat Greek yogurt

½ cup agave nectar

1 teaspoon vanilla extract

2 large eggs

1 cup cooked quinoa *(see recipe on page 238)*

½ cup chopped walnuts

❶ Preheat the oven to 350 degrees F. Lightly spray a 12-cup muffin tin with the oil spray.

❷ Sift the flour, salt, baking powder, and baking soda into a small bowl. Set aside.

❸ Put 1½ cups of the pichuberries in a blender and puree until smooth. Transfer the puree to a separate, large bowl along with the yogurt, agave, vanilla, and eggs. Whisk to combine.

❹ Gently whisk the dry ingredients into the wet ingredients, being careful not to overmix the batter.

❺ Slice the remaining ½ cup of pichuberries in half and add them to the batter along with the quinoa and walnuts. Stir to combine.

❻ Divide the batter among the twelve muffin cups. Bake for 25 minutes or until the muffins are golden.

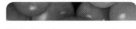

Pichuberries are a good source of vitamin E, vitamin A, vitamin P, and the B-complex vitamins B1, B6, and B12.

Per Serving: Kcal 277, Protein 8g, Carb 43g, Fat 9g, Sodium 536mg, Dietary Fiber 4g
Daily Values: Fiber 15%, Vit C 6%, Vit A 14%, Vit D 5 14%, Calcium 5%, Iron 10%

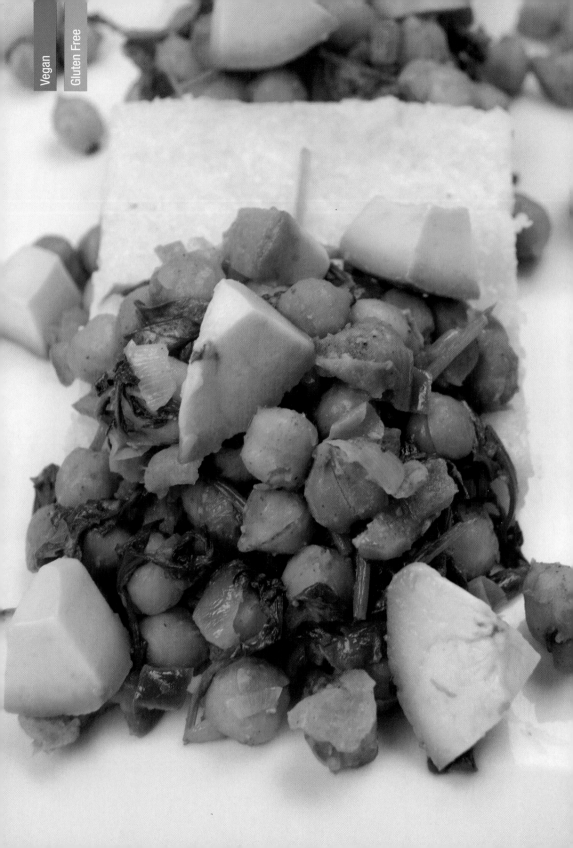

SAVORY POLENTA WITH CURRIED GARBANZO AND ARUGULA

Servings: 6 ♦ Serving size: 1 cup

Warm your heart and soul with this savory breakfast—perfect to make ahead.

1 cup polenta

3 to 4 cups water

Salt and pepper

1 tablespoon canola oil

1 medium red onion, chopped fine

2 cloves garlic, crushed

2 cans (*14 ounces each*) garbanzo beans, drained

1 teaspoon curry powder

1 teaspoon ground turmeric

4 cups arugula

Oil spray

❶ Put the polenta and 3 cups of the water into a deep, medium-size saucepan and bring to a boil over medium heat. Reduce heat and simmer gently, stirring frequently to prevent sticking. If the polenta thickens too quickly, add extra water as needed (up to 1 cup). The finished product should be very thick, and should cook for about 30 minutes. When the polenta is done, season it with salt and pepper to taste, and remove it from the heat.

❷ Coat a small sheet pan with a light layer of oil. Spread the polenta onto the pan in a one-inch layer and let cool.

❸ Heat 1 tablespoon of the oil in a large sauté pan over medium heat. When hot, add the onion and garlic. Sauté for 5 minutes or until the onions soften.

❹ Add the beans, curry, and turmeric to the pan. Sauté until hot and fragrant.

❺ Add the arugula and salt and pepper to taste. Cook just until the arugula is wilted.

❻ Slice the polenta into squares and spoon the curried garbanzo mixture over them. Serve warm.

NOTE: The polenta and curried garbanzo bean mixture will keep in the refrigerator for three to five days. Reheat both the polenta squares and garbanzo beans on a lightly oiled sauté pan until hot.

Per Serving: Kcal 197, Protein 5g, Carb 37g, Fat 3.5g, Sodium 206mg, Dietary Fiber 4g
Daily Values: Fiber 15%, Vit C 10%, Vit A 9%, Vit D 5 0%, Calcium 5%, Iron 12%

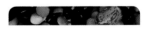

Beans are rich in fiber, folate, iron, magnesium, potassium, protein, and thiamine. Beans are also low in fat, making them great for weight loss.

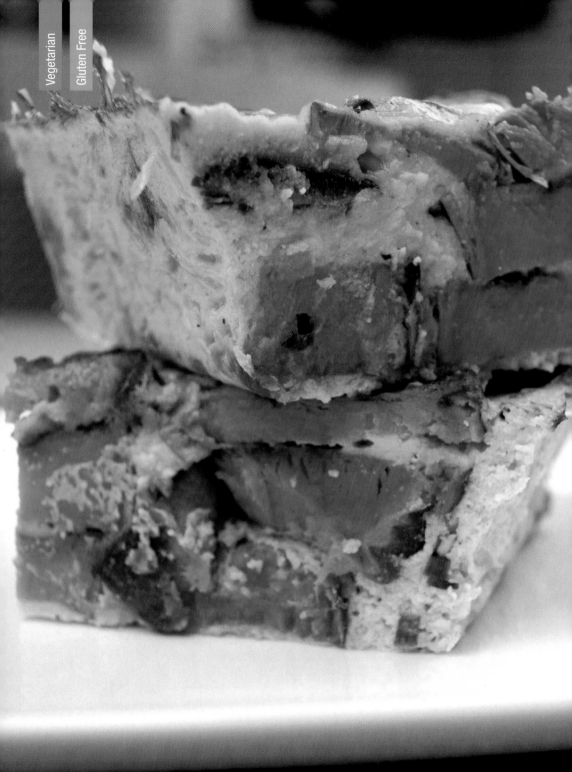

SWEET POTATO CRUSTLESS QUICHE

Servings: 8 ♦ Serving size: 1 cup

This fantastic quiche is a warm, savory, and satisfying breakfast the entire family will adore.

Coconut oil spray

2 large sweet potatoes *(about 2½ pounds),* sliced into ½-inch rounds

4 eggs

1 cup low-fat milk

1 cup low-fat ricotta cheese

¼ teaspoon salt

¼ teaspoon pepper

¼ teaspoon smoked paprika

Pinch of nutmeg

¼ cup chopped chives

❶ Preheat the oven to 400 degrees F. Lightly spray a sheet pan with the coconut oil.

❷ Place the sweet potato slices on the sheet pan and spray them with a thin layer of the coconut oil. Bake for 20 to 25 minutes until tender but not too browned. Let them cool.

❸ Lightly spray a 9 × 5–inch casserole dish with the coconut oil. Layer the sweet potato slices in the dish to form three to four loosely packed layers.

❹ Put the eggs, milk, ricotta, spices, and chives in a medium bowl and whisk to combine. Pour the egg mixture over the sweet potatoes, giving it time to fill in the gaps.

❺ Bake for 30 to 40 minutes until the center is just barely set. Serve warm.

Sweet potatoes are very high in beta-carotene, calcium, iron, and vitamins A and C. The vitamin A content far exceeds daily requirements.

Per Serving: Kcal 215, Protein 10g, Carb 32g, Fat 5.5g, Sodium 237.5mg, Dietary Fiber 4.5g
Daily Values: Fiber 17%, Vit C 7%, Vit A 410%, Vit D 5 6%, Calcium 18%, Iron 8%

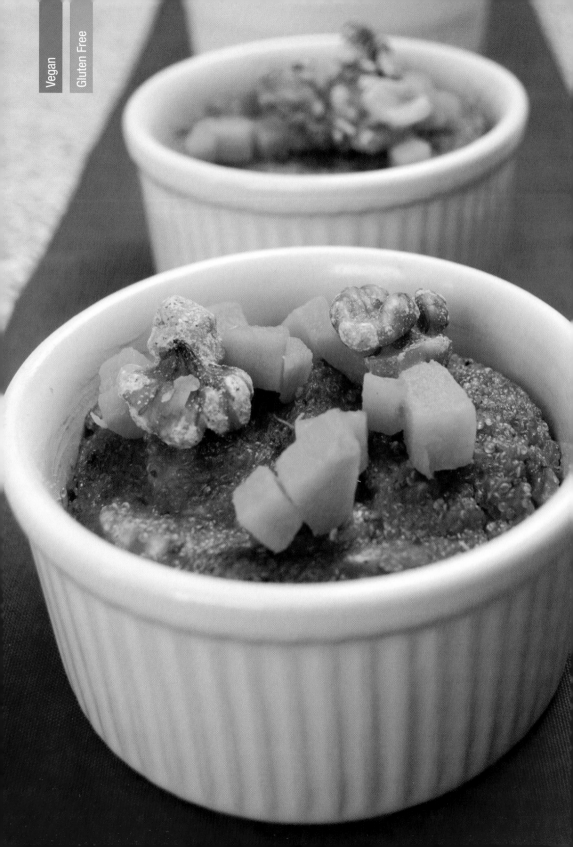

SWEET POTATO KIWICHA BREAKFAST BAKE

Servings: 6 ♦ Serving size: 1⅓ cups

1. Lightly spray a small casserole dish (or six personal-size ramekins) with cooking oil and set aside.

2. Put the sweet potato cubes in a medium saucepan with enough water to cover by an inch. Bring to a boil over medium-high heat and simmer for about 5 minutes until the sweet potatoes are tender. Drain them in a colander and set aside.

3. Put the kiwicha and the water in the saucepan. Bring to a boil over high heat and then reduce heat to a simmer. Cover and cook for 15 minutes or until all of the water has been absorbed.

4. Heat the oven to 350 degrees F.

5. Put the sweet potatoes and the banana in a medium bowl. Using a potato masher or fork, mash to combine.

6. Add the cooked kiwicha, almond milk, chia seeds, vanilla, cinnamon, nutmeg, and agave syrup to the bowl and mix to combine. Season with salt to taste.

7. Transfer the kiwicha mixture to the casserole dish (or ramekins) and bake uncovered for 20 minutes. After 20 minutes, change the oven setting to "broil" and cook for a few minutes to crisp the top, being careful not to burn it.

8. Serve warm topped with toasted walnuts.

Oil spray

1 large sweet potato, peeled and cubed *(1-inch cubes)*

1 cup kiwicha

2 cups water

2 bananas

1 cup unsweetened almond milk

2 tablespoons chia seeds

4 teaspoons vanilla extract

2 teaspoons ground cinnamon

¼ teaspoon ground nutmeg

2 tablespoons agave syrup

Salt

½ cup walnuts, toasted

The fiber from chia seeds can absorb large amounts of water and expands in the stomach, which should increase fullness and slow the absorption of food.

Per Serving: Kcal 319, Protein 8g, Carb 49.5g, Fat 10.5g, Sodium 67mg, Dietary Fiber 8g
Daily Values: Fiber 33%, Vit C 11%, Vit A 128%, Vit D 5 4%, Calcium 12%, Iron 21%

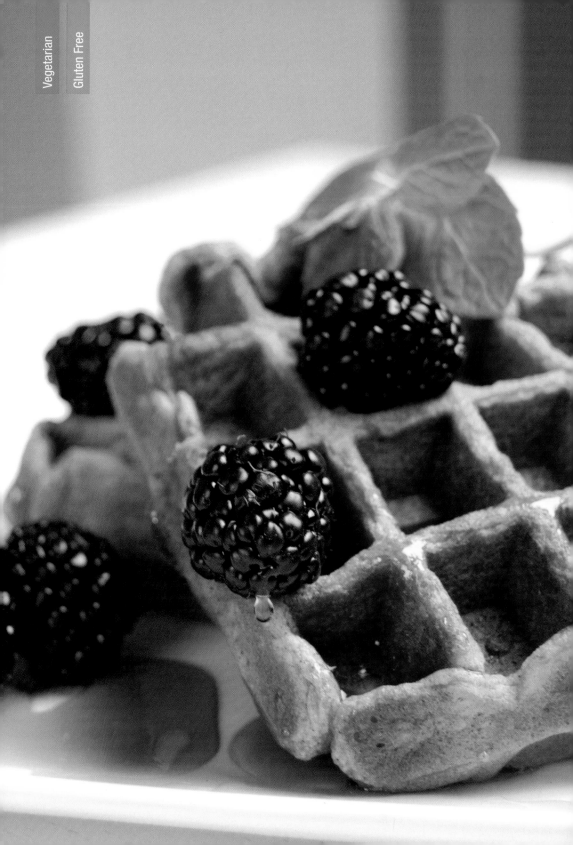

SWEET POTATO WAFFLES

Servings: 8 ◆ Serving size: 1 waffle (about 4 inches x 4 inches)

These are perfect for a traditional Sunday family breakfast, and they're kid-approved, too. This waffle recipe is so delicious and naturally sweet, you don't even need to add syrup—an extra bonus for minimizing your waistline.

❶ Preheat a waffle iron.

❷ Put the sweet potatoes, milk, 2 of the egg yolks, and the brown sugar in a large bowl and whisk to combine. Add the flour, baking powder, cinnamon, and salt to the wet ingredients. Whisk to combine.

❸ Put all the egg whites in a separate large bowl. Using a handheld electric blender with the whisk attachment, or a standard mixer, whip the whites until they form soft peaks.

❹ Gently fold the whipped whites into the sweet potato batter.

❺ When the waffle iron is hot, spray it with a coat of oil. Make the waffles according to the waffle iron instructions.

2 cups mashed boiled sweet potatoes *(see recipe on page 234)*

1 cup low-fat milk

6 eggs, separated

¼ cup packed brown sugar

1¾ cups oat flour, sifted

1 tablespoon baking powder

2 teaspoons ground cinnamon

½ teaspoon salt

Oil spray

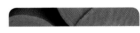

Sweet potatoes are rich in beta-carotene, a powerful antioxidant that has been shown to prevent oxidative damage, which can help prevent both cancer and cardiovascular disease.

Per Serving: Kcal 234, Protein 9.5g, Carb 39.5g, Fat 4.5g, Sodium 378.5mg, Dietary Fiber 4g
Daily Values: Fiber 17%, Vit C 18%, Vit A 261%, Vit D 5 5%, Calcium 12%, Iron 11%

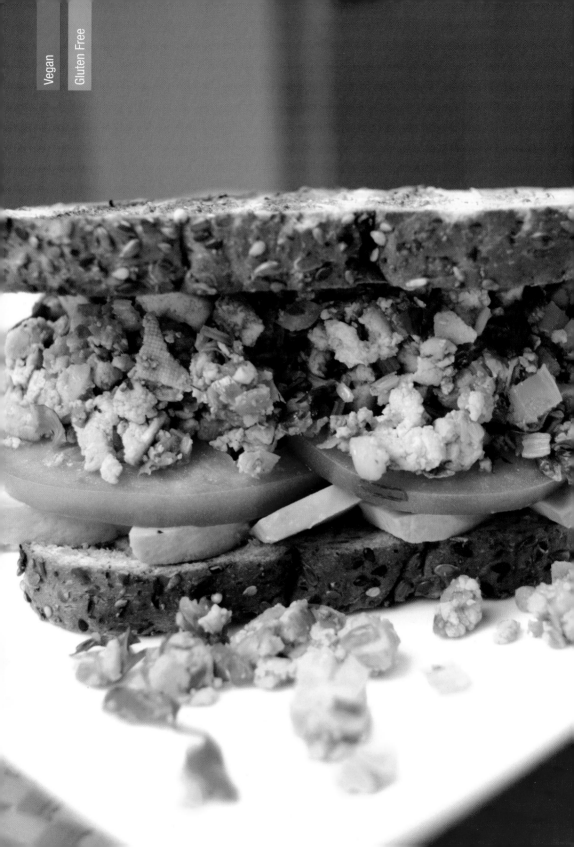

TOFU BREAKFAST SCRAMBLE

Servings: 4 ◆ Serving size: 1 cup

This mouthwatering scramble recipe comes to us from our colleague and chef, Chenoa Bol. Chenoa is a dear friend and a vegetarian, and she inspired me to create the vegetarian and vegan versions of the recipes in this book. Knowing how much of a food lover she is, I was shocked to hear she had never tried Peruvian cuisine. A lot of Peruvian dishes are made with some type of meat such as fish, chicken, or beef, so Chenoa had previously shied away from trying the food. Hearing this, I was inspired to cook for her, and I decided to make a vegetarian version of Ají de Gallina. Instead of using chicken, I used tempeh but with all the other classic ingredients of the dish. She was able to experience one of my favorite Peruvian dishes and instantly fell in love. This helped me realize that we can make alternative versions of the classic Peruvian dishes for everyone without losing the love, passion, and flavors of the original dishes. I've tried many tofu dishes over the years, but this was the first to arouse a true "wow" moment! Chenoa's use of spices and flavors were simply perfect!

1 tablespoon canola oil

1 package *(14 ounces)* firm tofu, drained and cut into 1-inch cubes

½ medium red onion, chopped very fine

1 large carrot, grated

1 large rib celery, chopped very fine

3 cloves garlic, crushed

1 tablespoon Bragg's Liquid Aminos *(or salt)*

¾ teaspoon ground turmeric

¾ teaspoon curry powder

¾ teaspoon ground cumin

¾ teaspoon ground smoked paprika

⅓ cup chopped cilantro

❶ Heat the oil in a sauté pan over medium heat. When the oil is hot, add the tofu, onion, carrot, and celery. Mash the tofu with a fork or potato masher as it is cooking until it is the desired consistency. Cook until the onions wilt.

❷ Season the tofu mixture with the garlic, Bragg's, turmeric, curry, cumin, and paprika.

❸ Cook until the tofu begins to dry out and brown. Turn off the heat and stir in the cilantro.

NOTE: Tofu scramble will keep in the refrigerator for three to five days and can be used to prepare additional breakfast sandwiches or wraps.

Per Serving: Kcal 150, Protein 11g, Carb 5g, Fat 10g, Sodium 209mg, Dietary Fiber 2g
Daily Values: Fiber 8%, Vit C 4%, Vit A 6%, Vit D 5 0%, Calcium 14%, Iron 13%

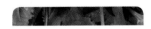

Cilantro is rich in beta-carotene, folic acid, niacin, riboflavin, vitamin A, and vitamin C and is a natural antioxidant. It's also a good source of calcium, iron, magnesium, manganese, and potassium.

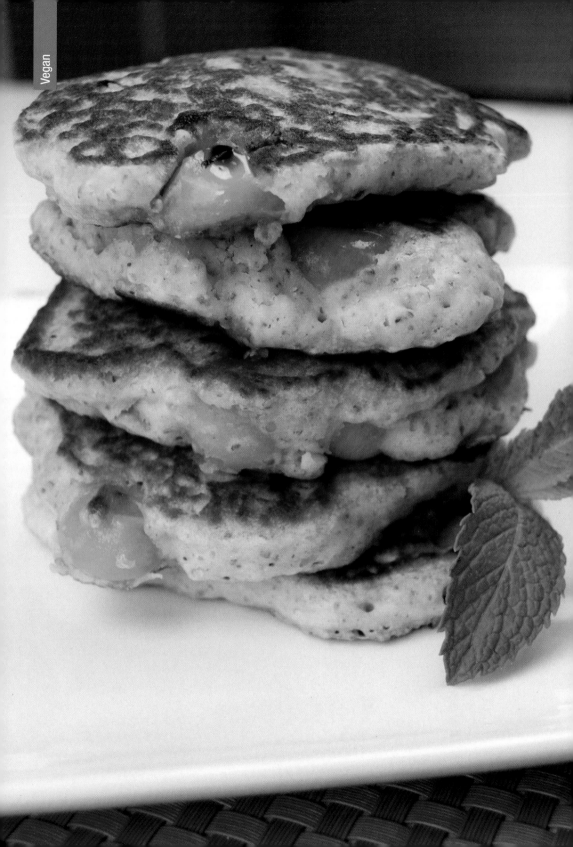

VEGAN PICHUBERRY PANCAKES

Servings: 8 ◆ Serving size: One 3-inch pancake

Enjoy these scrumptious pancakes during a relaxing weekend breakfast.

❶ Put the ground chia seeds and the water in a small bowl. Whisk to combine and set aside.

❷ Combine the flour, sugar, baking powder, baking soda, and salt in a large mixing bowl. Whisk to combine and set aside.

❸ Quickly whisk the melted coconut oil into the chia seed mixture. Once it's completely combined, add the milk, vinegar, and vanilla to the bowl. Mix thoroughly.

❹ Add the wet mixture to the dry mixture and whisk to combine, being careful not to overmix the batter. Gently fold in the pichuberries.

❺ Lightly coat a large sauté pan with the oil spray and place over medium heat. When the pan is hot, ladle about ½ cup of the batter per pancake into the pan. When the pancake begins to firm up and form small air bubbles on the surface, for 1 to 2 minutes, flip to cook the other side for another 1 to 2 minutes until golden. Lightly coat the pan with another layer of oil before cooking the next round of pancakes.

❻ Serve immediately.

Per Serving: Kcal 112.5, Protein 4g, Carb 18g, Fat 3g, Sodium 174mg, Dietary Fiber 2g
Daily Values: Fiber 7%, Vit C 4%, Vit A 6%, Vit D 5 7%, Calcium 3%, Iron 6%

4 teaspoons ground chia seeds

3 tablespoons water

1 cup all-purpose flour, sifted

1 teaspoon sugar

1 teaspoon baking powder

¼ teaspoon baking soda

¼ teaspoon salt

1 tablespoon coconut oil, melted

1 cup unsweetened almond milk

1 teaspoon apple cider vinegar

1 teaspoon vanilla extract

1 cup pichuberries, halved

Coconut oil spray

By eating only 3 ounces of this power fruit, you'll meet 37 percent of your daily required vitamin A, 13 percent of your required niacin, 18 percent of your recommended vitamin C, and 39 percent of your vitamin D requirement (percent of daily values are based on a 2,000-calorie diet).

VERY COCONUTTY KAÑIWA CEREAL

Servings: 6 ♦ Serving size: 1½ cups

2 cups quick-cooking rolled oats

½ cup kañiwa (or kiwicha or amaranth)

1 cup dried yacon slices (or dried apple slices)

1 cinnamon stick

¼ teaspoon salt

2 cups low-fat milk

4½ cups water

6 tablespoons unsweetened, shredded coconut

Enjoy a fiber-filled meal that is perfect for warming your heart and soul, and satisfying your belly. This dish is packed with incredible superfoods, amazing antioxidants, and outstanding vitamins.

❶ Put the oats, kañiwa, yacon, cinnamon stick, salt, milk, and water in a medium stockpot. Bring to a boil over medium heat, then reduce to low heat. Cook for 15 to 20 minutes, stirring constantly, to desired consistency.

❷ Top each serving with 1 tablespoon coconut before serving.

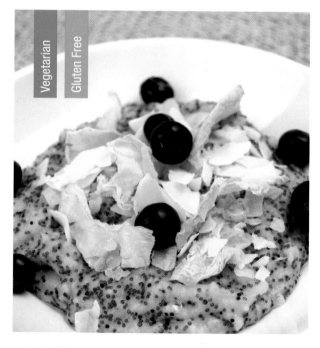

Vegetarian | Gluten Free

Combined with soluble fiber, yacon can make you feel fuller while you eat, which can help with weight loss. It slows absorption of sugars into the bloodstream.

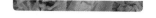

Per Serving: Kcal 269, Protein 10g, Carb 47g, Fat 5g, Sodium 177mg, Dietary Fiber 5g
Daily Values: Fiber 20%, Vit C 5%, Vit A 6%, Vit D 5 11%, Calcium 16%, Iron 28%

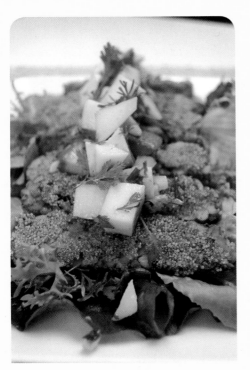

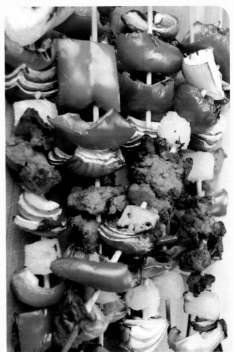

Main Dishes

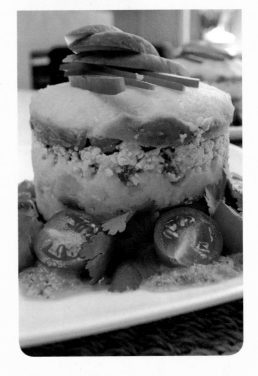

AJÍ DE TEMPEH
OVER ROASTED ZUCCHINI

Servings: 6 ◆ Serving size: 1 cup

Olive oil spray

6 large zucchinis

Salt and pepper

3 slices whole grain
bread, broken into
small pieces

2 cups vegetable broth

1 tablespoon canola oil

5 cloves garlic, sliced

1 medium white onion,
chopped

1 tablespoon ground
cumin

2 tablespoons ají
amarillo paste (or mild
chili paste)

1 teaspoon turmeric

2 teaspoons salt

2 teaspoons black
pepper

½ cup evaporated milk

2 blocks (8 ounces each)
tempeh, cut into strips

2 ounces walnut pieces

¼ cup shredded
Parmesan cheese

3 hard-boiled eggs,
halved*

*This is our vegetarian version of the classic Peruvian
meal ají de gallina.*

For the roasted zucchini:

❶ Preheat the oven to 400 degrees F. Lightly spray a
baking sheet with the oil spray.

❷ Slice each zucchini in half lengthwise. Place each
half on the baking sheet cut side up. Lightly coat
the halves with the oil spray and season with salt
and pepper to taste.

❸ Bake for 20 minutes until tender and lightly golden
around the edges.

For the ají de tempeh:

❶ Put the bread and the vegetable broth in a blender
or the bowl of a food processer and let it soak for
10 minutes.

❷ Meanwhile, heat the oil in a large sauté pan over
medium heat. When the oil is hot, add the garlic,
onion, cumin, ají, and turmeric and cook until
nicely browned, for about 5 minutes.

❸ Carefully transfer the onion mixture to the blender
or food processor with the bread and broth. Add
the salt, pepper, and evaporated milk. Puree to
form a smooth sauce.

❹ Transfer the sauce, along with the tempeh, to a
large sauté pan. Cook over medium-low heat for
5 to 10 minutes until the sauce thickens. Stir in the
walnuts and the Parmesan cheese.

❺ Serve the ají de tempeh on top of the roasted
zucchini and top with half of a hard-boiled egg.

*The hard-boiled eggs and roasted zucchini are not included in
the nutrient analysis.*

Per Serving: Kcal 383, Protein 23g, Carb 27g, Fat 23g, Sodium 1240mg, Dietary Fiber 3.5g
Daily Values: Fiber 14%, Vit C 5%, Vit A 2%, Vit D 5%, Calcium 29%, Iron 20%

ANDEAN GRAIN PILAF

Servings: 6 ◆ Serving size: ½ cup

You have heard of quinoa and kiwicha; now meet their sister, kañiwa. All of these three seeds are natives of the Andean region and used as highly nutritional food by the Incas. Try this delicious pilaf as your grain of choice for some complete protein and a power carbohydrate.

1 tablespoon olive oil

1 medium onion, diced

1 clove garlic, minced

1 tablespoon ají amarillo paste *(or mild chili paste)*

¼ cup quinoa

¼ cup kiwicha

¼ cup kañiwa

1½ cups vegetable broth

Salt and pepper

❶ Put the olive oil in a large sauté pan over medium heat. When hot, add the onion and garlic and sauté until soft and fragrant. Stir in the ají paste and cook for another minute.

❷ Place the grains, vegetable broth, salt, and pepper into a small saucepan. Bring to a boil and lower the heat to a simmer. Cover and cook until all of the water is absorbed, for 15 to 20 minutes. When done, fluff with a fork and set aside to cool.

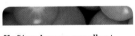

Kañiwa has an excellent nutrition profile. It contains 15 percent of protein per ¼ cup serving, 3 grams of fiber, and a wealth of antioxidants, zinc, iron, and calcium.

Per Serving: Kcal 113g, Protein 4g, Carb 17g, Fat 173g, Sodium 2mg, Dietary Fiber 9g
Daily Values: Fiber 11%, Vit C 1%, Vit A 4%, Vit D 5 0%, Calcium 3%, Iron 16%

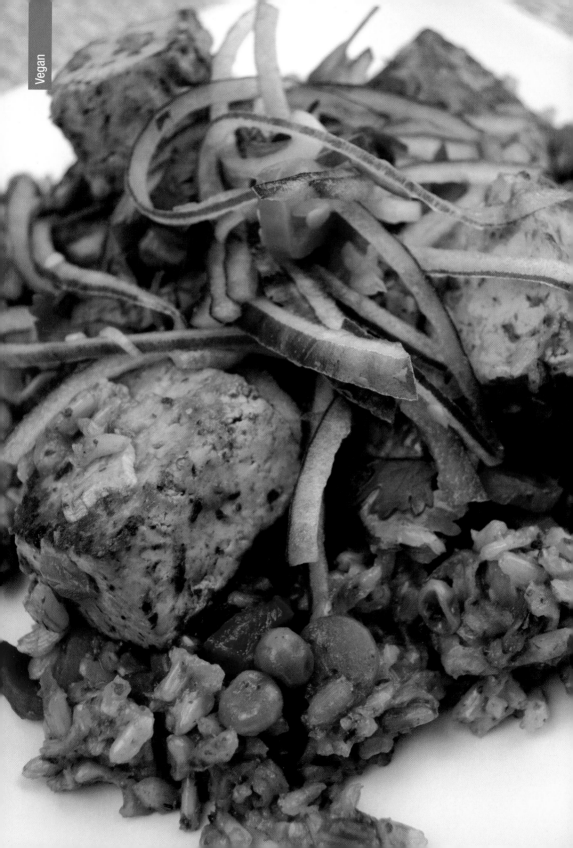

ARROZ CON TOFU

Servings: 6 ♦ Serving size: 1 cup

This recipe has the same flavors as the classic Peruvian dish arroz con pollo, but it is vegan so that everyone may enjoy it. Let the famous cilantro sauce wow your taste buds and bring a happy dance to your soul.

4 teaspoons canola oil

1 block *(14 ounces)* firm tofu, cut into 1½-inch pieces

1 tablespoon ají amarillo paste *(or mild chili paste)*

1 tablespoon ground cumin

Salt and pepper

3 cups vegetable stock

1 bunch cilantro, stems removed

1 large red onion, diced

4 cloves garlic, minced

1 large carrot, diced

2 large celery ribs, diced

1 medium red bell pepper, diced

1 cup brown rice

1 cup frozen peas

❶ Heat 2 teaspoons of the oil in a large sauté pan over medium heat. When the oil is hot, add the tofu, ají, and cumin and cook until nicely browned, for about 5 minutes. Season with salt and pepper to taste. Set aside.

❷ To prepare a cilantro broth, put the vegetable stock and cilantro in a blender and process until a smooth green liquid is formed.

❸ Heat the remaining oil in a medium-size stockpot over medium heat. When the oil is hot, add the onion, garlic, carrot, celery, and bell pepper and cook until fragrant, for about 5 minutes. Season with salt and pepper to taste.

❹ Add the cilantro broth, rice, and peas to the pot and stir to combine. Place the tofu on top of the rice mixture.

❺ Cover the pot and lower the temperature to a simmer. Cook for 40 to 50 minutes or until all of the water has been absorbed.

Per Serving: Kcal 243, Protein 10g, Carb 34g, Fat 18g, Sodium 555.5mg, Dietary Fiber 4.5g
Daily Values: Fiber 18%, Vit C 57%, Vit A 65%, Vit D 5 0%, Calcium 13%, Iron 12%

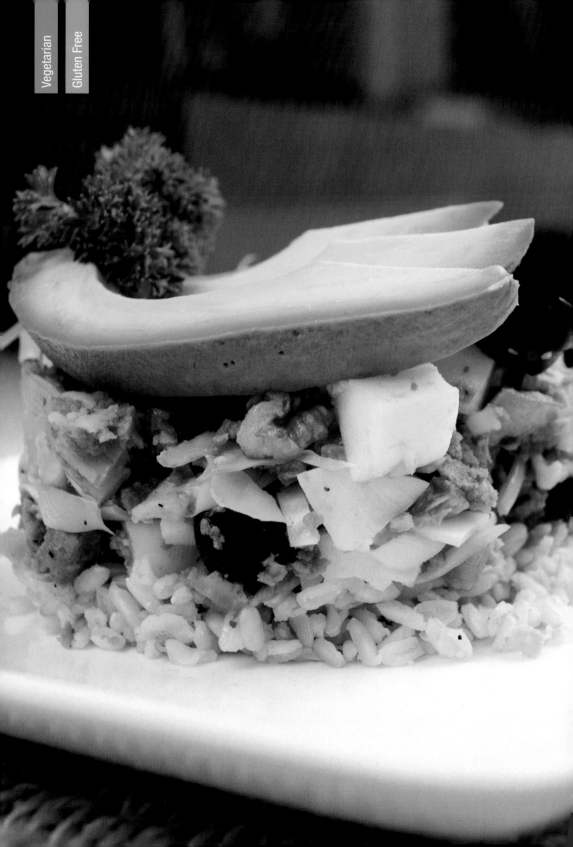

ARTICHOKE SEITAN MOLIDO

Servings: 6 ◆ Serving size: 1 cup

The inspiration for this dish comes from arroz tapado, which is a layer of rice, beef, eggs, and more rice on top. "Molido" means "ground." This is a vegetarian version of the dish using seitan for the protein and artichokes for the veggies. Serve this on top of rice or add it to any dish where you need a hearty filling.

2 boxes *(8 ounces each)* **seitan**

1 tablespoon olive oil

1 large yellow onion, diced

2 cloves garlic, minced

1 tablespoon ají amarillo paste *(or mild chili paste)*

1 can *(14 ounces)* **sliced black olives**

1 can *(14 ounces)* **artichoke hearts in water, drained and diced**

¼ cup walnut pieces

Salt and pepper

2 hard-boiled eggs, diced

❶ Put the seitan in the bowl of a food processor and pulse until coarsely ground. Set aside.

❷ Heat the oil in a large sauté pan over medium heat. When the oil is hot, add the onion and garlic and cook until fragrant, for about 2 minutes. Add the ají and ground seitan and cook for another 5 to 7 minutes or until browned and fragrant.

❸ Add the olives, artichokes, and walnuts to the pan and cook until just heated through. Season with salt and pepper to taste. Remove from the heat and stir in the hard-boiled eggs.

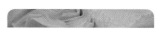

Artichokes are a great source of dietary fiber, which means they can help lower the risk of developing heart disease, stroke, hypertension, and diabetes. Fiber also improves blood sugar levels and insulin sensitivity in nondiabetic and diabetic individuals.

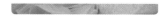

Per Serving: Kcal 272.5, Protein 23.5g, Carb 16.5g, Fat 14g, Sodium 1395mg, Dietary Fiber 7g
Daily Values: Fiber 29%, Vit C 9%, Vit A 7%, Vit D 5 2%, Calcium 11%, Iron 23%

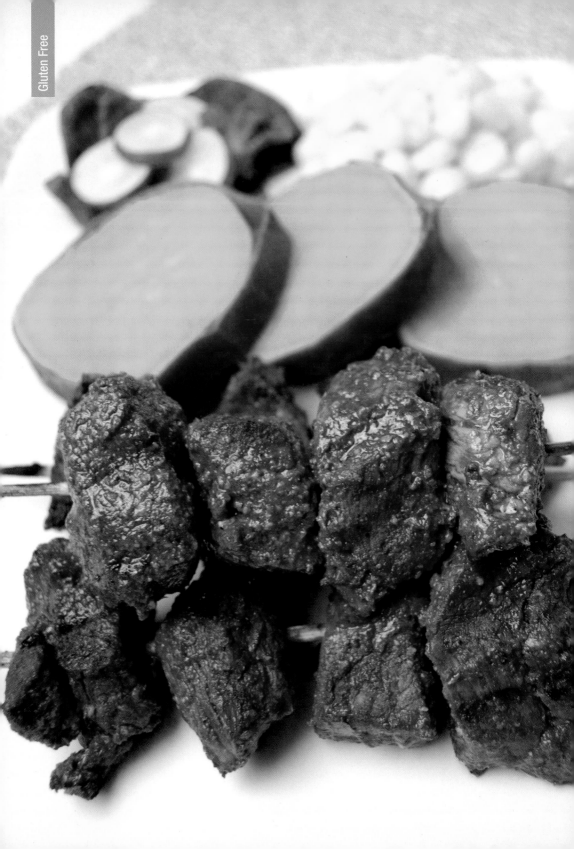

BEEF ANTICUCHOS

Servings: 10 ♦ Serving size: 1 skewer

Anticuchos are traditionally made out of beef hearts, and the best versions are found on the street. Peruvians enjoy this dish when out and about. Here we use sirloin steak and keep all the traditional flavors of anticuchos without the added fat or cholesterol. Hello, health!

12 cloves garlic, crushed

1 tablespoon ground cumin

¼ cup ají panca paste *(or mild chili paste)*

¼ cup white wine vinegar

1 teaspoon salt

1 tablespoon ground black pepper

1 tablespoon canola oil

2 pounds steak *(sirloin or tenderloin)*, cut into 1½-inch pieces

Wooden skewers

❶ Place the wooden skewers in a casserole dish and fill the dish with water to cover. Let them soak for 30 to 60 minutes before using.

❷ Combine the garlic, cumin, ají, vinegar, salt, pepper, and oil in a large, shallow bowl. Whip with a fork to create a smooth, homogeneous mixture. Add the steak to the marinade and toss to coat. Let it marinate for 60 minutes at room temperature or overnight in the refrigerator.

❸ Divide the marinated meat among ten wooden skewers, making sure they have lots of sauce on them.

❹ Heat your grill according to the manufacturer's instructions. Grill the skewers, turning them as necessary until they are lightly charred. Remove and eat warm.

Per Serving: Kcal 214, Protein 18g, Carb 2g, Fat 9.5g, Sodium 396mg, Dietary Fiber 2g
Daily Values: Fiber 2%, Vit C 2%, Vit A 0%, Vit D 5 3%, Calcium 3%, Iron 11%

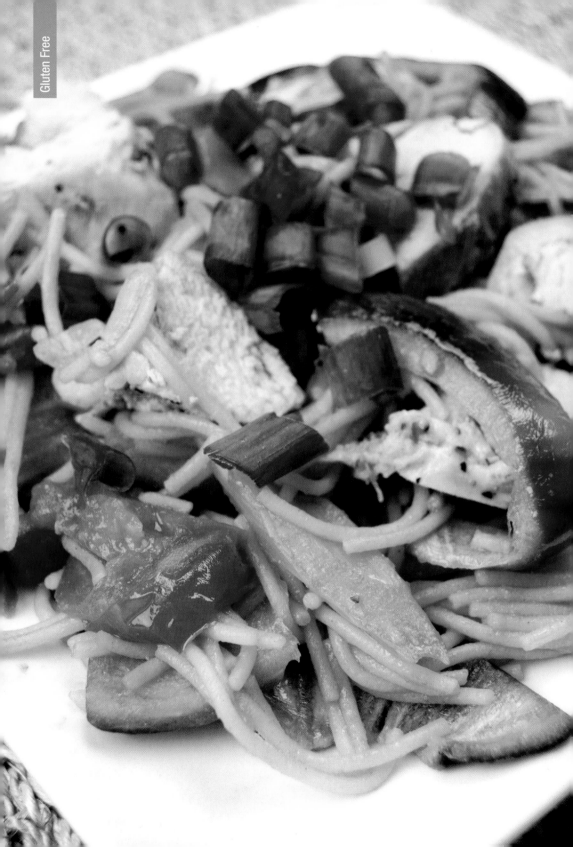

CHICKEN TALLARIN SALTADO

Servings: 5 ◆ Serving size: 2 cups

Tallarin saltado is a common Asian-inspired Peruvian dish that typically uses noodles. To accommodate gluten-free needs, we used another Peruvian superfood, quinoa, for all to enjoy.

❶ Heat the oil in a large sauté pan or wok over medium-high heat. Add the onion, celery, ginger, soy sauce, and vinegar to the pan. Cook for 2 to 3 minutes.

❷ Add the tomatoes, chicken, and scallions to the pan and stir to combine. Add the spaghetti. Cook until just heated through. Season with salt and pepper to taste.

1 tablespoon canola oil

1 large red onion, cut into strips

3 large celery ribs, cut into strips

1 teaspoon minced ginger

1 tablespoon low-sodium, gluten-free soy sauce

1 tablespoon white vinegar

3 medium tomatoes, cut into wedges

1 pound Weekend Oregano Roasted Chicken (*see recipe on page 152*), cubed

4 scallions, chopped

3½ cups cooked quinoa spaghetti (*about 8 ounces dry pasta*)

Salt and pepper

Per Serving: Kcal 334.5, Protein 24g, Carb 46g, Fat 6.5g, Sodium 687.5mg, Dietary Fiber 6g
Daily Values: Fiber 25%, Vit C 31%, Vit A 20%, Vit D 5 0%, Calcium 8%, Iron 20%

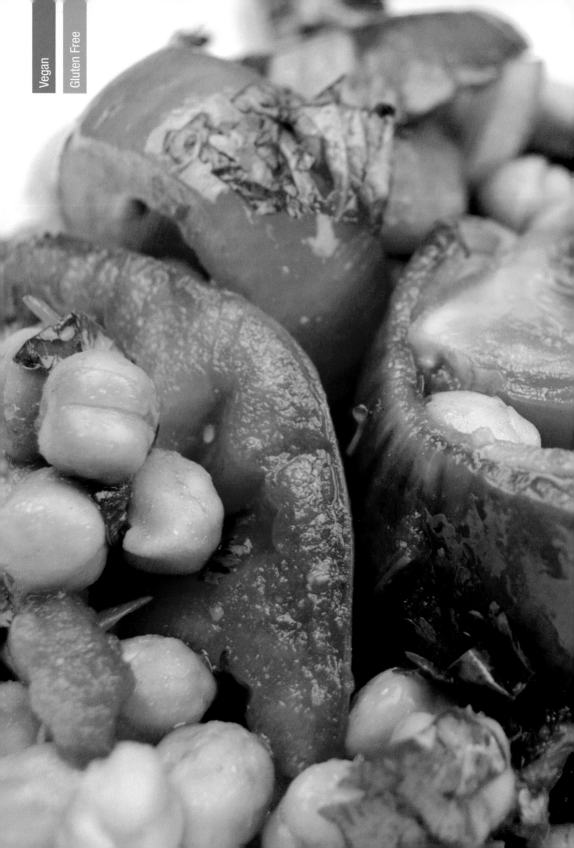

GARBANZO SALTADO

Servings: 5 ◆ Serving size: 1 cup

This is another fusion recipe inspired by the national classic Peruvian dish lomo saltado. This vegan version of the Asian-fused meal is extremely flavorful and exquisite.

1 tablespoon canola oil

2 cans *(15 ounces each)* garbanzo beans, drained

2 medium red onions, cut into strips

1 clove garlic, minced

1 tablespoon ají amarillo paste *(or mild chili paste)*

2 tablespoons balsamic vinegar

3 tablespoons low-sodium soy sauce

2 teaspoons ground cumin

2 tomatoes, cut into strips

Handful of fresh cilantro, chopped

❶ Heat the oil in a large sauté pan or wok over medium-high heat. Once the oil is hot, add the garbanzo beans, onions, garlic, ají, vinegar, soy sauce, and cumin to the pan. Cook for 3 to 5 minutes until the onions are fragrant but still hold their shape.

❷ Add the tomatoes and cook for 1 to 2 minutes longer. Remove the pan from the heat and add the cilantro. Stir to combine.

Per Serving: Kcal 274, Protein 10g, Carb 47.5g, Fat 5g, Sodium 917.5mg, Dietary Fiber 9g
Daily Values: Fiber 36%, Vit C 28%, Vit A 28%, Vit D 5 0%, Calcium 9%, Iron 15%

GARLIC BUTTER BEANS À LA PARMESAN

Servings: 8 ♦ Serving size: 1 cup

2 cups butter beans

1 tablespoon olive oil

1 medium yellow onion, diced

4 cloves garlic, sliced

1 tablespoon oregano

8 cups vegetable stock

1 cup dry sherry

Salt and pepper

½ cup grated Parmesan cheese

My mom used to make a dish using butter beans, called "pallares" in Spanish. This dish is inspired by my mom. I love her cooking! She tasted my version, said I did her justice, and gave me her blessing to share this dish with you. Buen provecho!

❶ Put the beans in a stockpot and cover them with 3 inches of water. Let them soak for 4 hours. Drain the beans in a colander, discarding the water.

❷ Transfer the beans back to the stockpot and cover with 3 inches of water. Bring them to a boil over medium heat. Drain the beans in a colander, discarding the water (this process helps remove the oxalates in beans that are responsible for gastrointestinal discomfort).

❸ Using the same pot, heat the oil over medium heat. When the oil is hot, add the onions, garlic, and oregano. Sauté until the onions begin to soften.

❹ Add the beans, stock, and sherry to the pot and bring to a boil. Season the beans with salt and pepper to taste. Cover, reduce heat, and cook at a simmer for about an hour or until the beans are soft. Stir in the Parmesan cheese. Serve warm.

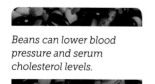

Beans can lower blood pressure and serum cholesterol levels.

Per Serving: Kcal 188, Protein 9g, Carb 16g, Fat 6g, Sodium 874.5mg, Dietary Fiber 3.5g
Daily Values: Fiber 14%, Vit C 3%, Vit A 2%, Vit D 5 1%, Calcium 22%, Iron 10%

GRILLED SALMON

Servings: 4 ♦ Serving size: 4 ounces

This recipe is a basic way to grill salmon for any occasion.

1 pound salmon with skin

1. Place the salmon, skin side down, in a casserole dish. Cover with the garlic, lemon juice, and salt and pepper to taste. Let the salmon marinate at room temperature for 30 minutes.

4 cloves garlic, crushed

2. Meanwhile, heat your grill according to the manufacturer's instructions.

3 tablespoons lemon juice

3. Grill the salmon, turning as necessary until the fish turns opaque and flakes when pulled apart with a fork. Serve immediately.

Salt and pepper

Per Serving: Kcal 244.5, Protein 26.5g, Carb 2g, Fat 15g, Sodium 987mg, Dietary Fiber 0g
Daily Values: Fiber 0%, Vit C 10%, Vit A 1%, Vit D 5 13%, Calcium 7%, Iron 4%

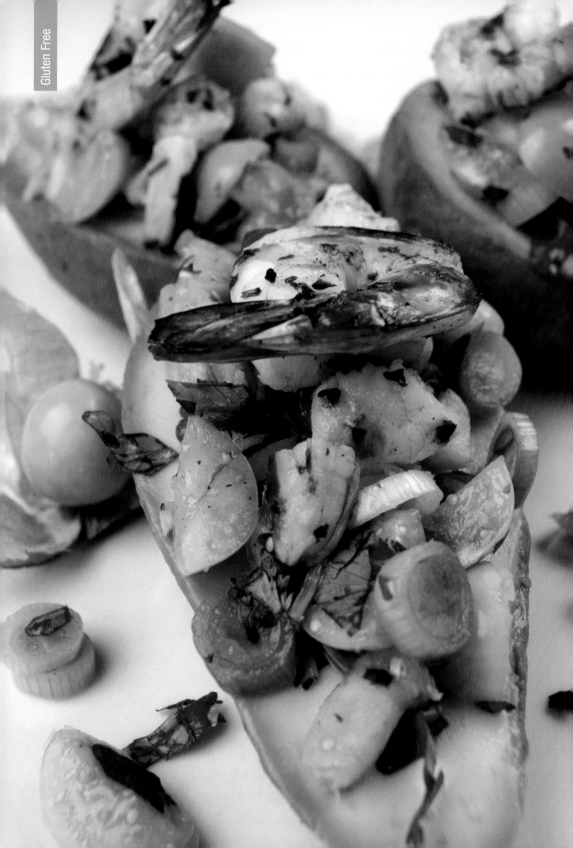

GRILLED SHRIMP-STUFFED AVOCADO

Servings: 4 ◆ Serving size: ½ stuffed avocado

Use the scooped-out avocado halves as a bowl to serve the delectable shrimp ceviche. It's a delicious and beautiful treat in one perfect package.

2 cloves garlic, crushed

1 tablespoon olive oil

6 tablespoons lime juice

Salt

8 ounces fresh shrimp, cleaned

2 green onions, thinly sliced

⅓ cup chopped cilantro

1 cup pichuberries, quartered

2 avocados

❶ Make a marinade by combining the garlic, oil, 3 tablespoons of the lime juice, and the salt, to taste, in a medium bowl. Add the shrimp and mix thoroughly to coat. Let the shrimp marinate at room temperature for 30 minutes.

❷ In the meantime, carefully cut the avocados in half so you can use the scooped-out halves for serving the ceviche. Remove the pits, score the flesh into cubes, and scoop it into a medium-size bowl. Add the onions, cilantro, remaining lime juice, and pichuberries and set aside.

❸ Heat your grill according to the manufacturer's instructions. Grill the shrimp for 2 to 3 minutes on each side, turning as necessary until they are lightly charred. Remove from the grill and let cool.

❹ Chop the shrimp into bite-size pieces and add them to the bowl with the avocados. Toss to combine.

❺ Distribute the filling among the avocado halves and eat that day.

Avocados are rich in essential nutrients, including fiber, folic acid, potassium, and vitamins B and E. They are high in antioxidants, carotenoids, lutein, and tocopherols. They are also low in cholesterol and low in sodium.

Per Serving: Kcal 234, Protein 14g, Carb 14g, Fat 15g, Sodium 108.5mg, Dietary Fiber 5g
Daily Values: Fiber 21%, Vit C 33%, Vit A 20%, Vit D 5 35%, Calcium 5%, Iron 11%

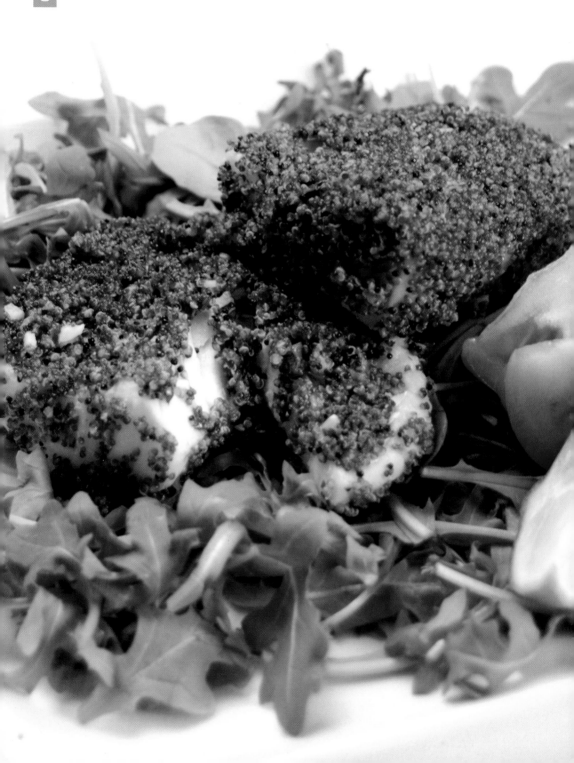

KAÑIWA CRUSTED COD

Servings: 2 ♦ Serving size: 3 ounces of cod

For the kañiwa:

❶ Put the kañiwa, water, and salt in a small saucepan. Bring to a boil and lower the heat to a simmer. Cover and cook until all of the water is absorbed, about 15 minutes. When done, fluff with a fork and set aside to cool.

For the cod:

❶ Put the olive oil, garlic, cilantro, and lime juice in a shallow bowl. Add salt and pepper to taste and mix to combine.

❷ Place the fillets in the marinade and let them sit for 5 minutes. Flip them over and let them marinate for another 5 minutes.

❸ Put the kañiwa on a large plate. Roll the marinated fillets in the kañiwa, pressing it into the flesh until both sides are coated.

❹ Spray a large sauté pan with cooking oil and heat over medium heat. When hot, add the fillets. Cook for about 5 minutes on one side; flip over and cook the other side.

❺ Place the fillets on a platter and serve with fresh lime wedges.

For the kañiwa:

¼ cup kañiwa

½ cup water

¼ teaspoon salt

For the cod:

1 tablespoon olive oil

1 clove garlic, crushed

1 tablespoon chopped cilantro

2 teaspoons lime juice

Salt and pepper

6 ounces cod fillets

Oil spray

Lime wedges

¼ cup of dry kañiwa provides 60 percent of the recommended daily value for iron at 11mg.

Per Serving: Kcal 216, Protein 19g, Carb 17g, Fat 7g, Sodium 685mg, Dietary Fiber 2g
Daily Values: Fiber 7%, Vit C 9%, Vit A 2%, Vit D 5 9%, Calcium 4%, Iron 33%

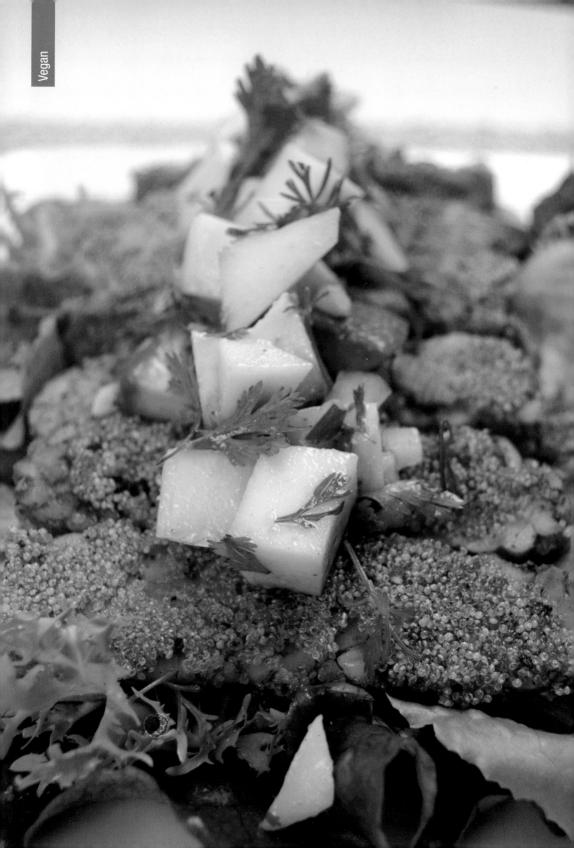

KIWICHA CRUSTED TEMPEH

Servings: 8 ♦ Serving size: 1 slice

Experience a true fusion of Peruvian flavors for a vegan palate with this crunchy, protein-packed dish. Prep the tempeh on a weekend and enjoy it easily throughout the week. Serve over a salad or any grain dish.

2 tablespoons canola oil

½ teaspoon ground cumin

½ teaspoon lemon pepper

½ teaspoon ground paprika

½ teaspoon garlic powder

Salt

16 ounces *(1 package)* **tempeh, sliced ½-inch thick lengthwise**

1 cup popped kiwicha *(see recipe on page 220)*

Oil spray

❶ Put the oil, cumin, lemon pepper, paprika, garlic powder, and salt in a small bowl. Mix to combine.

❷ Dip the tempeh slices in the spiced oil mixture. Then dip the slices in the popped kiwicha. Place the slices on a sheet pan; dip and coat the remaining slices.

❸ Spray a large sauté pan with the canola oil and heat over medium-high heat. When the pan is hot, place half of the tempeh slices into the pan to form a single layer. Let them cook until lightly browned, for 2 to 3 minutes. Flip the slices to cook the other side. Repeat the process with the remaining tempeh slices.

NOTE: Tempeh is best eaten right away; however, it will keep in the refrigerator for three to five days.

Kiwicha contains fiber, and it's a complete source of protein, meaning it contains all nine essential amino acids. This is a great option for vegetarians and vegans seeking plant-based protein sources.

Per Serving: Kcal 157.5, Protein 11g, Carb 8.5g, Fat 10g, Sodium 26mg, Dietary Fiber 0.5g
Daily Values: Fiber 2%, Vit C 1%, Vit A 1%, Vit D 5 0%, Calcium 7%, Iron 11%

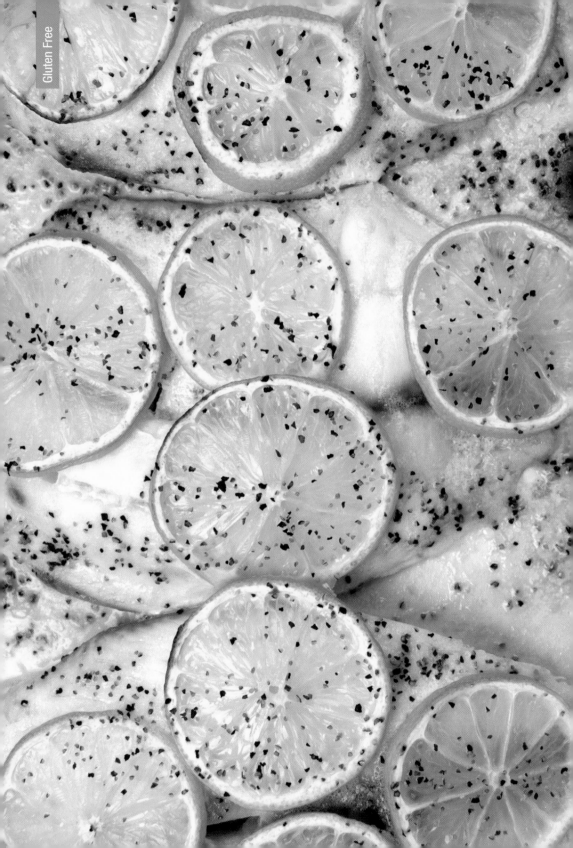

Gluten Free

LEMON-ROASTED FISH

Servings: 4 ♦ Serving Size: 1 fillet

This is a basic recipe for roasting fish—quick, easy, and simple.

❶ Preheat the oven to 375 degrees F.

❷ Place the fillets in a roasting pan and coat them with the lemon juice, oil, and salt and pepper.

❸ Slice the whole lemon into thin rounds, and remove the seeds from each slice. Distribute the slices equally among the fish fillets.

❹ Roast the fillets for 15 to 25 minutes (depending on the thickness of the fillets) until the fish is white and flakes when pulled apart with a fork. Serve immediately.

4 fillets white fish
(sea bass, tilapia, or sol)

Juice of 1 lemon
(about 3 tablespoons)

1 lemon, whole

2 tablespoons olive oil

Salt and pepper

Per Serving: Kcal 109, Protein 25g, Carb 6g, Fat 9.5g, Sodium 92mg, Dietary Fiber 2.5g
Daily Values: Fiber 10%, Vit C 69%, Vit A 0%, Vit D 5 0%, Calcium 5%, Iron 4%

LENTIL-QUINOA MASACHAKUY

Servings: 4 ◆ Serving size: 1¼ cups

1 tablespoon canola oil

1 medium onion, diced

1 clove garlic, minced

1 tablespoon ají
amarillo paste *(or mild
chili paste)*

1 teaspoon ground
cumin

2 cups cooked quinoa
(see recipe on page 238)

2 cups cooked lentils
(see recipe on page 238)

Salt and pepper

Handful of fresh
cilantro, chopped

*"Masachakuy" means "marriage" in the Andean
language of Quechua. With this succulent meal,
we married lentils and quinoa to provide a perfect
love affair in your mouth.*

❶ Heat the oil in a large sauté pan over medium
heat. When the oil is hot, add the onion and
garlic. Sauté until soft and fragrant. Stir in the
ají and cumin and cook for another minute.

❷ Add the quinoa and the lentils to the pan and
cook until heated through. Season with salt
and pepper to taste. Toss with the fresh cilantro
before serving.

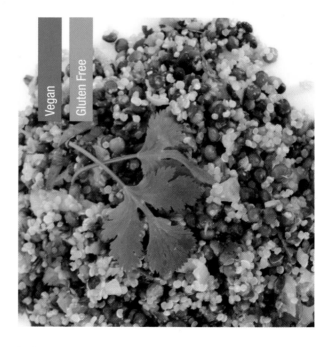

Vegan | Gluten Free

Per Serving: Kcal 232.5, Protein 12g, Carb 36.5g, Fat 5g, Sodium 79.5mg,
Dietary Fiber 10g
Daily Values: Fiber 40%, Vit C 9%, Vit A 3%, Vit D 5 0%, Calcium 5%, Iron 28%

LOMO SALTADO

Servings: 4 ◆ Serving size: 1½ cups

Lomo saltado is a traditional Peruvian dish that is a true infusion of Asian married to Peruvian cuisine in this nationwide classic meal.

❶ Heat the oil in a large sauté pan over medium-high heat. Put the beef tri-tip in the pan, along with the cumin and salt and pepper to taste. Cook the meat until it is nicely browned.

❷ Add the onions, garlic, ají, and vinegar to the pan. Cook for 2 to 3 minutes and then turn off the heat. Add the tomatoes, cilantro, and soy sauce to the pan and stir to combine.

❸ Top the lomo saltado with sweet potato fries before serving.

*The sweet potato fries are not included in the serving size or nutrient analysis.

2 tablespoons canola oil

1 pound beef tri-tip, thinly sliced into strips

2 teaspoons ground cumin

Salt and pepper

2 medium red onions, cut into strips

1 clove garlic, minced

1 tablespoon ají amarillo paste *(or mild chili paste)*

2 tablespoons balsamic vinegar

2 large tomatoes, sliced into wedges

Handful of fresh cilantro, chopped

3 tablespoons low-sodium soy sauce

1 recipe Baked Sweet Potato Fries *(see recipe on page 213)**

Per Serving: Kcal 297, Protein 25.5g, Carb 12g, Fat 16g, Sodium 589mg, Dietary Fiber 2g
Daily Values: Fiber 8%, Vit C 20%, Vit A 12%, Vit D 5 0%, Calcium 6%, Iron 13

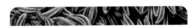

Just two teaspoons of cumin contain 15.5 percent of your recommended daily intake of iron.

Vegan

Gluten Free

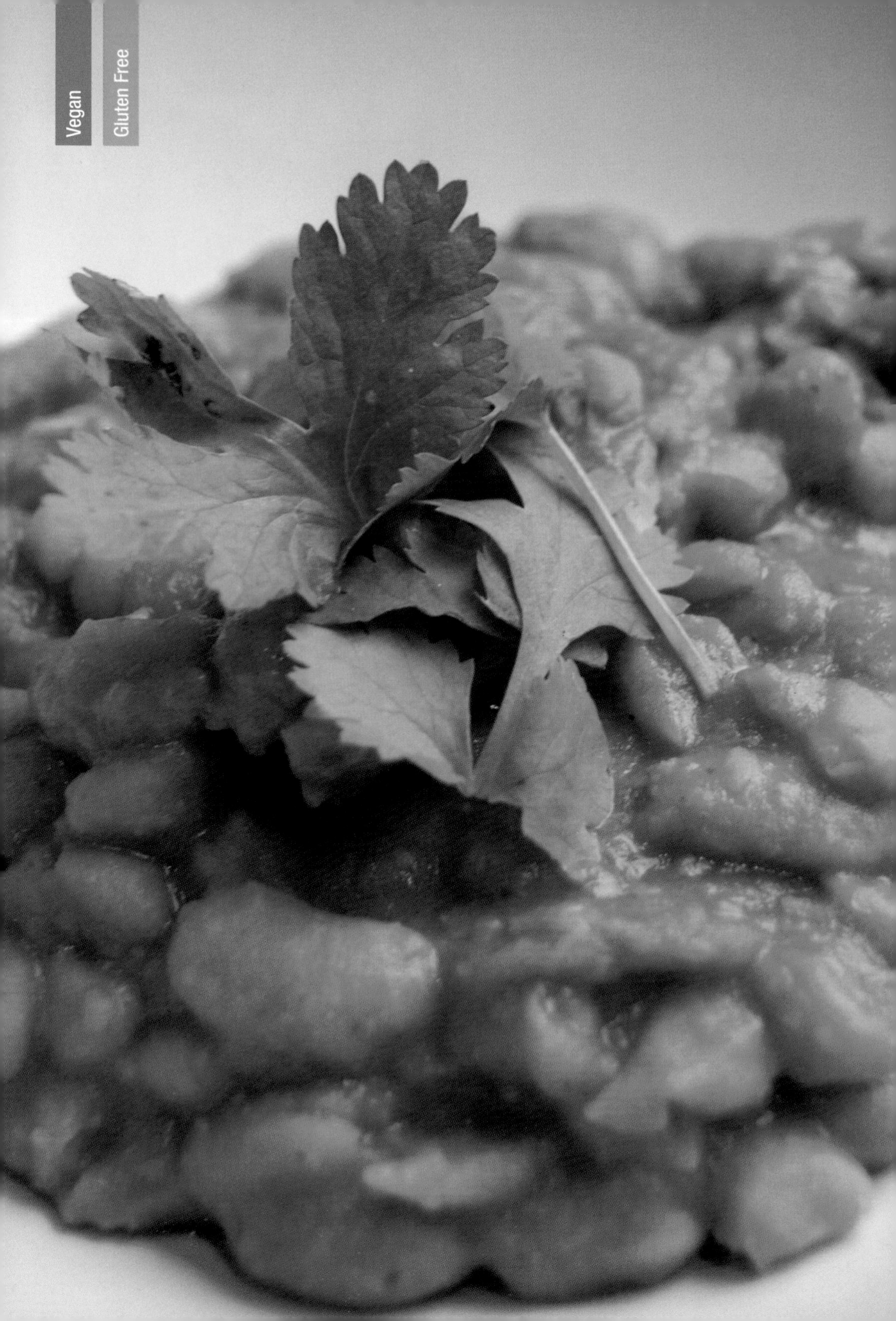

PERUVIAN BEANS À LA CILANTRO

Servings: 4 ♦ Serving size: 1½ cups

The cilantro sauce for this dish is used in many of the classical Peruvian cuisines such as arroz con pollo and beef seco. Inspired by the sauce, we fused these traditional flavors with a vegan version of pure satisfaction.

1 pound canary beans

2 tablespoons canola oil

1 medium red onion, chopped

2 cloves garlic, minced

1 tablespoon ají amarillo paste *(or mild chili paste)*

1 teaspoon ground cumin

1 bunch cilantro

4 cups vegetable stock

Salt and pepper

❶ Put the beans in a stockpot and cover with 3 inches of water. Let them soak for 4 hours. Drain the beans in a colander, discarding the water.

❷ Transfer the beans back into the stockpot and cover with 3 inches of water. Bring to a boil over medium heat. Drain the beans in a colander, discarding the water (this process helps remove the oxalates in beans, which are responsible for gastrointestinal discomfort).

❸ Transfer the beans back into the stockpot and set aside.

❹ Put the oil in a medium-size sauté pan over medium heat. When hot, prepare the *aderezo* (seasoning) by adding the onion, garlic, ají, and cumin to the pot. Sauté the mixture until soft and fragrant. Add the aderezo to the pot with the beans.

❺ Put the cilantro and stock in a blender. Puree until smooth and transfer to the pot of beans.

❻ Bring the beans, aderezo, and cilantro mixture to a boil over medium heat. Season with salt and pepper to taste. Cover, reduce the heat, and cook the beans at a simmer for about 1 hour or until the beans are soft. Serve warm.

In addition to beans, cilantro, which is also rich in iron, supports red blood cell production.

Per Serving: Kcal 307, Protein 7g, Carb 47g, Fat 8g, Sodium 295mg, Dietary Fiber 3.5g
Daily Values: Fiber 15%, Vit C 7%, Vit A 11%, Vit D 5 0%, Calcium 4%, Iron 3%

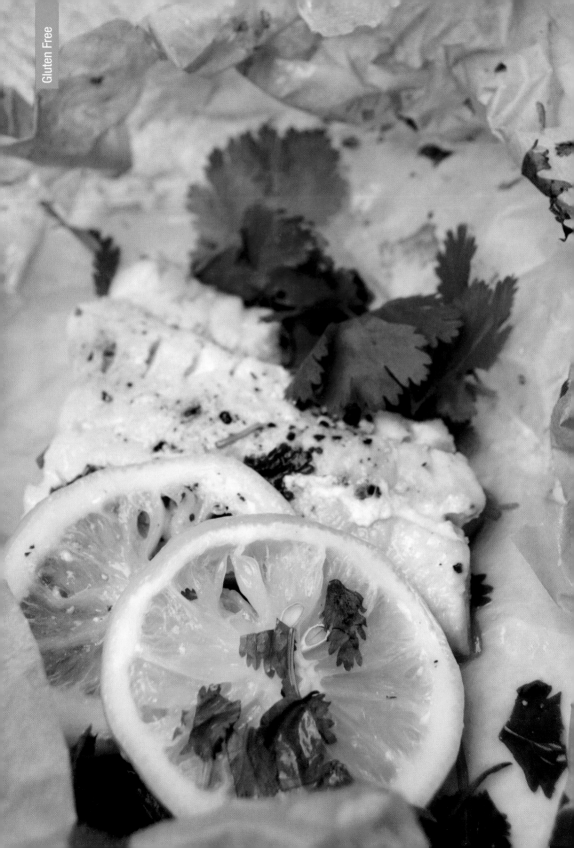

PERUVIAN FISH PACKETS

Servings: 4 ♦ Serving size: One 4-ounce fish packet

Looking for a meal in less than thirty minutes? This recipe is perfect for a quick and easy dinner with minimal cleanup and very few dishes to wash.

Four 8-inch squares aluminum foil

Four 8-inch squares parchment paper

¼ cup lemon juice

2 teaspoons olive oil

1 cup white wine

1 pound Alaskan cod or other white fish

Salt and pepper

1 lemon, sliced into ⅛-inch rounds

¼ cup chopped cilantro

❶ Preheat the oven to 400 degrees F. Place four squares of aluminum foil on a baking sheet, leaving about one inch of space between them. Top each piece of foil with a square of parchment paper and set aside.

❷ Put the lemon juice, oil, and wine in a small bowl and mix to combine.

❸ Cut the fish into four 4-ounce portions, placing one portion on each of the parchment squares. Gently pull up the sides of the foil to create a bowl around each piece of fish.

❹ Distribute the lemon mixture evenly among the fish packets. Season with salt and pepper to taste. Top each fish packet with lemon slices and cilantro.

❺ Carefully pull the edges of each foil packet to the center to form a sealed package. Bake for 20 to 25 minutes or to desired doneness. Eat immediately.

Studies show that cilantro has a protective effect on the cells of the heart, helping to prevent heart attacks and oxidative damage.

Per Serving: Kcal 230, Protein 22g, Carb 6.5g, Fat 9g, Sodium 641mg, Dietary Fiber 1.5g
Daily Values: Fiber 1.5%, Vit C 47%, Vit A 4%, Vit D 5 0%, Calcium 5%, Iron 4%

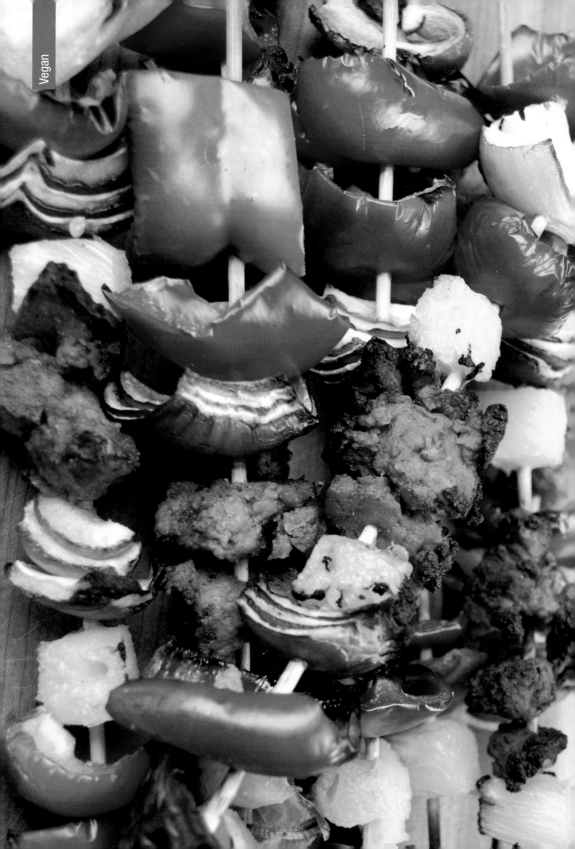

PERUVIAN SPICED SEITAN AND VEGGIE SHISH KEBABS

Servings: 8 ♦ Serving size: 1 skewer

Barbecue time! These Peruvian shish kebabs will wake up your taste buds and no one will miss the meat. Marinate the seitan overnight to enhance the flavor and add extra love.

❶ Place the wooden skewers in a casserole dish and fill with water to cover. Let them soak for 30 to 60 minutes before using.

❷ Combine the soy sauce, lime juice, garlic, cumin, and ají in a large, shallow bowl. Mix with a fork to create a smooth, homogeneous mixture. Add seitan cubes to the marinade and toss to coat. Let them marinate for 60 minutes at room temperature (or overnight in the refrigerator).

❸ Heat your grill according to the manufacturer's instructions.

❹ Drain the marinade from the seitan and reserve it to use as a dipping sauce for the cooked skewers (keep it in the refrigerator until ready to use).

❺ To make the skewers, place equal amounts of marinated seitan, bell pepper, onion, and pineapple on each skewer.

❻ Once the grill is hot, grill the skewers, turning them as necessary until they form a light char. Remove and eat warm or cold.

Wooden skewers

¼ cup soy sauce

¼ cup lime juice

1 clove garlic, minced

1 tablespoon ground cumin

1 tablespoon ají amarillo paste *(or mild chili paste)*

8 ounces *(1 package)* seitan, drained and cut into 1-inch cubes

1 medium green bell pepper, cut into 1-inch pieces

1 medium red bell pepper, cut into 1-inch pieces

1 small red onion, cut into 1-inch pieces

1 can *(20 ounces)* pineapple chunks in juice (not syrup), drained

Per Serving: Kcal 106, Protein 8g, Carb 16.5g, Fat 1g, Sodium 678.5mg, Dietary Fiber 2g
Daily Values: Fiber 8%, Vit C 69%, Vit A 11%, Vit D 5 0%, Calcium 2%, Iron 6%

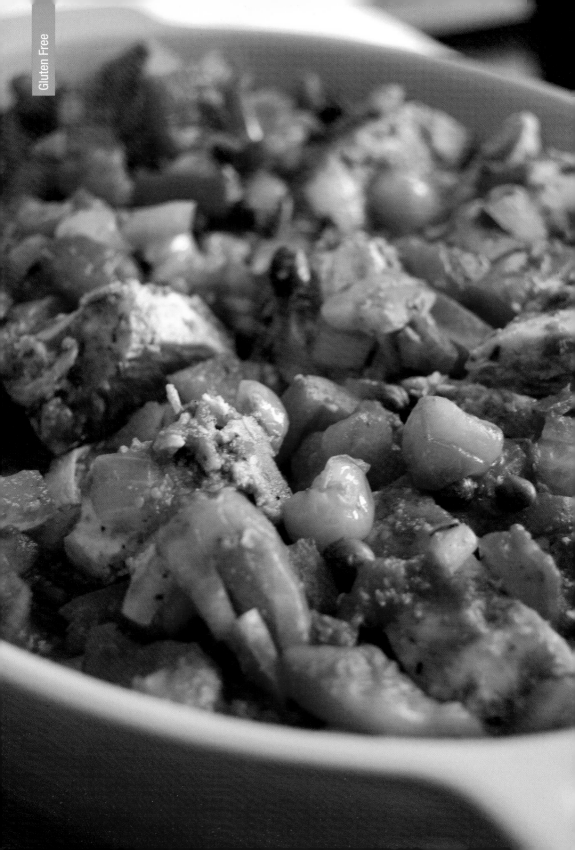

PICHUBERRY CHICKEN CACCIATORE

Servings: 4 ♦ Serving size: 1½ cups

The word cacciatore means "hunter" in Italian, and the phrase "alla cacciatora" refers to a meal prepared "hunter-style," thus referencing a classic meal preparation using some of Italy's most rustic ingredients: meat, tomatoes, onions, herbs, bell peppers, and red wine. As a lover of cacciatore as well as Peruvian cuisine, I thought, "Why not marry the two?" While utilizing the common preparation and ingredients of cacciatore, my addition of pichuberries created the perfect Peruvian touch, contributing sweet yet tart flavor notes. Delicious!

2 tablespoons olive oil

1 medium bell pepper, diced into ½-inch pieces

1 small onion, diced into ½-inch pieces

3 garlic cloves, minced

3 Roma tomatoes, diced into ½-inch pieces

1½ cups tomato sauce

¾ cup red wine

2 tablespoons capers, drained

1 cup pichuberries, halved

2 tablespoons oregano

Salt and pepper

1 pound Weekend Oregano Roasted Chicken (*see recipe on page 152*)

❶ Heat the oil in a large sauté pan over medium heat. When hot, add the bell pepper, onion, and garlic. Sauté for 5 minutes until soft and fragrant.

❷ Add the tomatoes, tomato sauce, wine, capers, pichuberries, and oregano to the pan. Add salt and pepper to taste. Sauté for 10 to 15 minutes until tender. Add the roasted chicken to the pan and cook just until heated through.

Pichuberries are a powerful antiaging agent because their vitamin C content and withanolides help reduce oxidation and inflammation.

Per Serving: Kcal 321, Protein 27g, Carb 22g, Fat 11g, Sodium 1310.5mg, Dietary Fiber 5g
Daily Values: Fiber 21%, Vit C 92%, Vit A 41%, Vit D 5 13%, Calcium 11%, Iron 20%

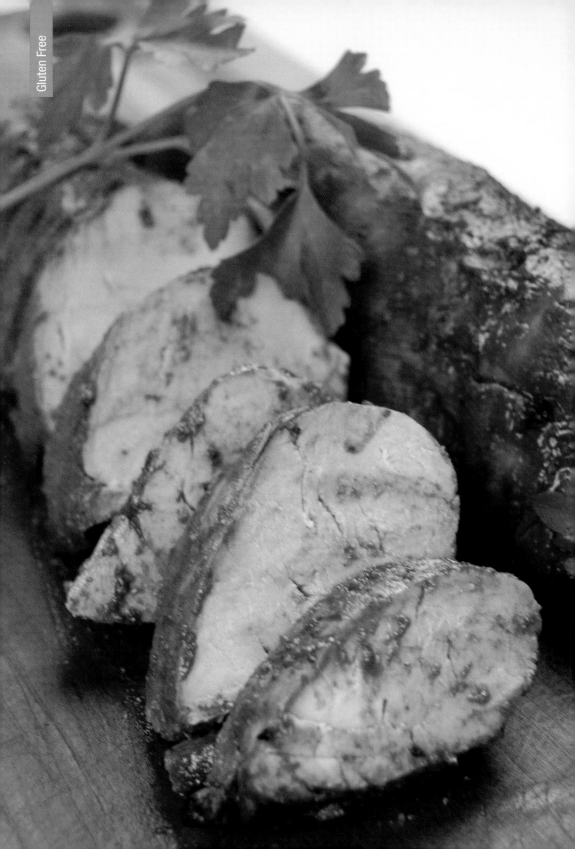

PORK TENDERLOIN WITH PERUVIAN SPICE RUB

Servings: 8 ♦ Serving size: 4 ounces

Ají, the most common chili pepper in Peru, provides a unique and wonderful flavor to the pork. With the combination of cumin, turmeric, and ají, you'll have a powerhouse of anti-inflammatory, antioxidant benefits to reboot the entire family.

2 tablespoons canola oil

1 teaspoon cumin

1 teaspoon turmeric

¼ cup ají panca paste *(or mild chili paste)*

3 cloves garlic, crushed

2 pounds pork tenderloin

❶ Combine the oil, cumin, turmeric, ají, and garlic in a small bowl. Stir to form a spice paste.

❷ Place the pork tenderloin in a small roasting pan and coat with the spice rub, making sure to cover the entire surface. Let it marinate at room temperature for 30 minutes.

❸ Preheat the oven to 400 degrees F.

❹ Roast the pork tenderloin for 20 minutes or until desired doneness. Let it cool slightly before slicing and serving.

The yellow pigment of turmeric, called curcumin, is thought to be the primary pharmacological agent in turmeric. Curcumin's anti-inflammatory effects have been shown to be as comparably potent as hydrocortisone, as well as over-the-counter anti-inflammatory agents such as Motrin.

Per Serving: Kcal 196.5, Protein 25g, Carb 1g, Fat 9.5g, Sodium 192mg, Dietary Fiber 0.5g
Daily Values: Fiber 1%, Vit C 1%, Vit A 0%, Vit D 5 2%, Calcium 3%, Iron 6%

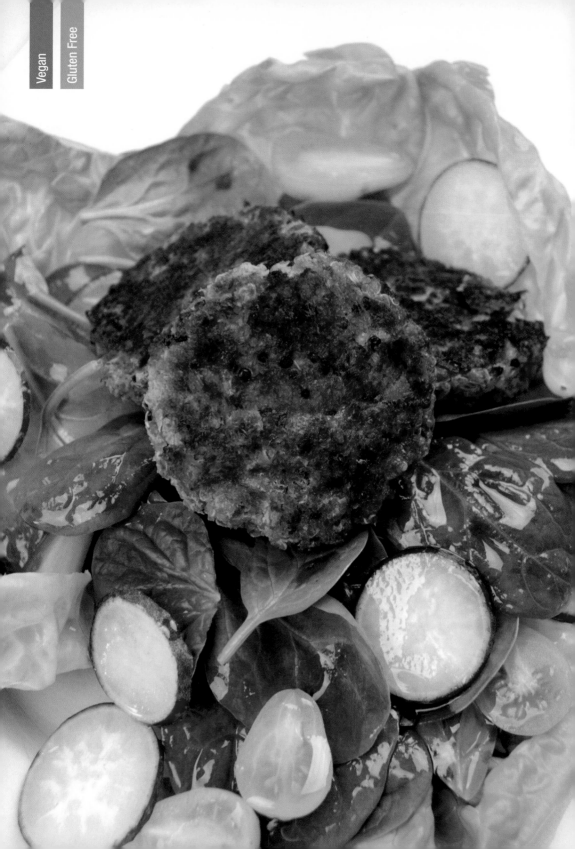

QUINOA CANNELLINI BEAN CROQUETTES

Servings: 12 ◆ Serving size: One 2-inch croquette

Croquettes are usually fried and breaded and are found worldwide in multiple cuisines. Our croquettes keep all of the flavor in a baked version combined with power protein foods to keep you satisfied and strong.

❶ Preheat the oven to 450 degrees F.

❷ Put the cannellini beans in the bowl of a food processor and process until very smooth, adding a little water if necessary. Remove the bean puree and put it in a medium bowl with the quinoa. Set aside.

❸ Heat the oil in a medium-size sauté pan over medium-low heat. When the oil is hot, add the onion, garlic, and carrot. Sauté until soft, fragrant, and lightly browned. Let cool.

❹ Put the vegetable mixture in the bowl of a food processor and process until coarse. Add the mixture to the bowl with the quinoa and bean puree. Mix to combine.

❺ Flavor the mixture with cumin and salt and pepper to taste.

❻ Lightly spray a sheet pan with oil. Divide the mixture into twelve portions. Roll each portion into a ball and place it on the baking sheet. Gently pat each ball into a 2-inch circle. Spray each croquette with a thin layer of the oil.

❼ Bake for 20 to 25 minutes until golden. Remove from the oven and eat warm or at room temperature.

Per Serving: Kcal 70.5, Protein 3.5g, Carb 11g, Fat 2g, Sodium 119.5mg, Dietary Fiber 3g
Daily Values: Fiber 11%, Vit C 1%, Vit A 17%, Vit D 5 0%, Calcium 3%, Iron 5%

1 can *(15 ounces)* cannellini beans, drained

1 cup cooked quinoa *(see recipe on page 238)*

1 tablespoon canola oil

½ medium onion, chopped

1 clove garlic, minced

1 medium carrot, chopped

1 tablespoon ground cumin

Salt and pepper

Oil spray

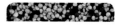

Quinoa has a low glycemic index of 35. For people suffering from diabetes, quinoa is a great carbohydrate source because it affects blood sugar at a slow rate once eaten.

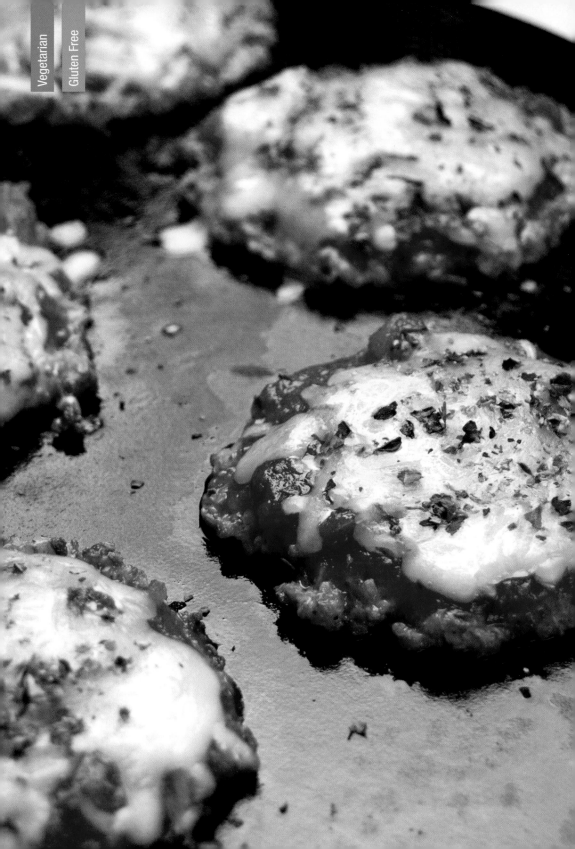

QUINOA PARMESAN PIZZETTES

Servings: 8 ♦ Serving Size: One 4-inch pizzette

Who doesn't like pizza? Here is a guilt-free version of pizza that uses quinoa for the crust, so you get your protein and fiber while nourishing your soul. These are perfect for the entire family to enjoy and very kid-friendly. For a gluten-free take, substitute the all-purpose flour with a gluten-free flour.

1 cup cooked quinoa *(see recipe on page 238)*

¼ cup all-purpose flour, sifted

½ cup liquid egg whites

½ cup grated Parmesan cheese

1 tablespoon dried oregano

1 teaspoon salt

1 teaspoon pepper

Oil spray

1 cup marinara sauce

8 ounces shredded mozzarella cheese

❶ Preheat a pizza stone in a 400 degree F oven.

❷ Put the quinoa, flour, egg whites, Parmesan cheese, oregano, and salt and pepper in a medium-size bowl and mix to combine.

❸ Pull the hot pizza stone out of the oven and spray it with a thin, even layer of oil. Divide the batter into eight portions. Pat each portion of batter into a 3-inch circle on the pizza stone, leaving an inch or two of space between the pizzettes. Bake for 15 to 20 minutes until golden.

❹ Remove the pizzettes from the oven and top each with about 2 tablespoons of marinara sauce and a handful of cheese. Return them to the oven and bake for 3 to 5 minutes longer, until the cheese is melted and bubbly. Cool slightly before eating.

Per Serving: Kcal 162.5, Protein 12.5g, Carb 11g, Fat 7.5g, Sodium 715mg, Dietary Fiber 2g
Daily Values: Fiber 9%, Vit C 1%, Vit A 7%, Vit D 5 0%, Calcium 31%, Iron 6%

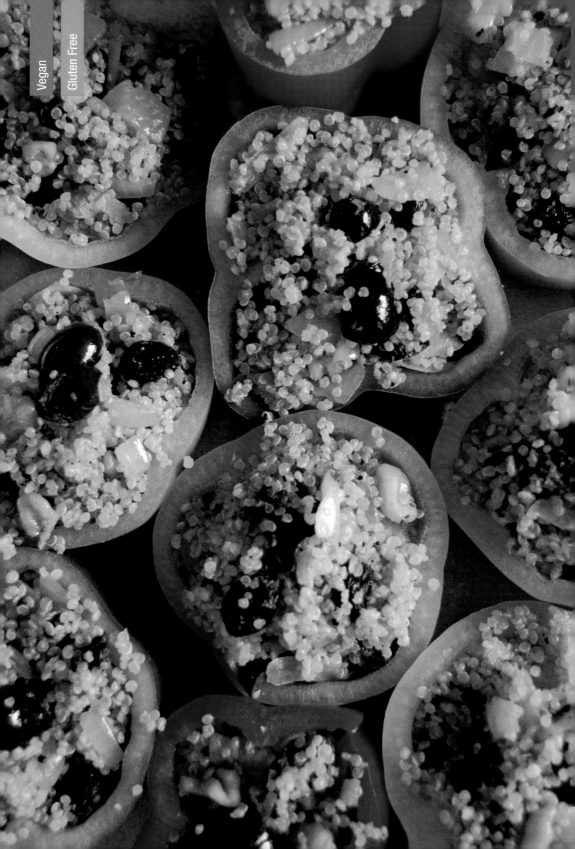

QUINOA-STUFFED BELL PEPPERS

Servings: 6 ♦ Serving size: ½ bell pepper

Using tricolor quinoa and tricolor bell peppers not only gives you a rainbow of health benefits but also a rainbow of visual appeal to wow your friends and family at your next potluck.

❶ Preheat the oven to 350 degrees F. Spray a medium-size baking dish with the oil spray.

❷ Heat the oil in a large sauté pan over medium heat. When hot, add the onion and garlic to the pan. Sauté for 1 to 2 minutes.

❸ Add the olives, raisins, and walnuts. Cook until lightly browned and fragrant.

❹ Combine the sautéed mixture with the quinoa. Flavor with salt and pepper to taste.

❺ Divide the quinoa mixture among the bell pepper halves. Place them in the baking dish and cover with foil.

❻ Bake for 45 to 60 minutes until the peppers are tender.

Oil spray

1 tablespoon oil of choice

½ medium onion, chopped fine

3 cloves garlic, crushed

1 cup whole, pitted olives, sliced

¼ cup raisins

¼ cup chopped walnuts

1½ cups cooked tricolor quinoa (*see recipe on page 238*)

Salt and pepper

3 large bell peppers, halved

Per Serving: Kcal 172, Protein 4g, Carb 21g, Fat 9g, Sodium 202mg, Dietary Fiber 4g
Daily Values: Fiber 15%, Vit C 82%, Vit A 6%, Vit D 5 0%, Calcium 5%, Iron 11%

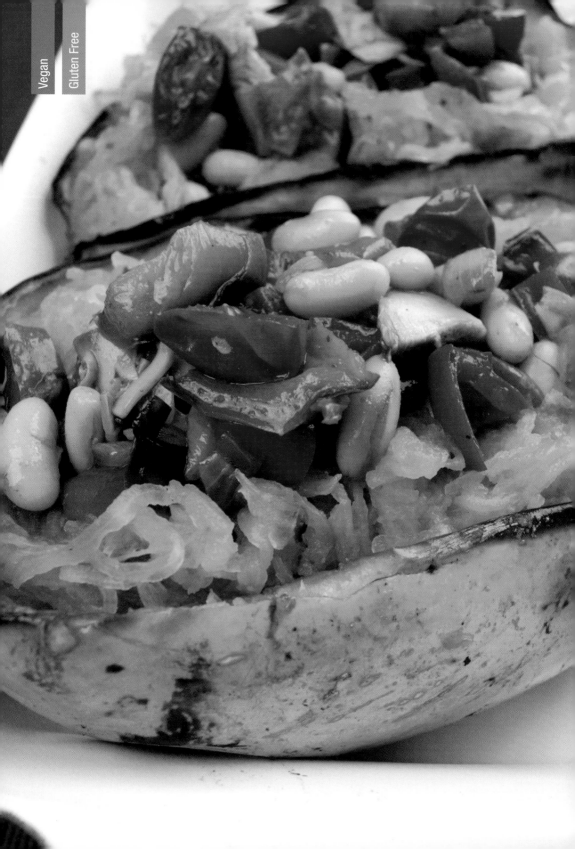

ROASTED SPAGHETTI SQUASH PRIMAVERA

Servings: 4 ♦ Serving size: ¼ squash, filled

Serve this amazing dish using the rind of the spaghetti squash as a bowl. Experience a burst of flavor with a rustic appeal from the organic food bowl.

❶ Preheat the oven to 425 degrees F. Lightly spray a baking sheet with oil.

❷ Place the spaghetti squash halves, cut side down, on the baking sheet. Cover them with the foil and bake for 45 to 60 minutes. Remove from the oven and let cool.

❸ While the squash is baking, heat the oil in a large sauté pan over medium heat. When hot, add the tomatoes, peppers, and onions to the pan. Sauté for 1 to 2 minutes or until the onion has softened. Turn off the heat and let cool.

❹ Once the squash and veggies have cooled, transfer the veggies to a medium bowl and add the beans, artichoke hearts, and sacha inchi oil. Season with the salt, pepper, and basil to taste. Mix to combine.

❺ Using a spoon, scrape the cooked squash into the bowl with the veggies. Toss to combine.

❻ Fill each squash shell with half of the mixture and serve.

Oil spray

1 spaghetti squash, cut in half lengthwise

2 teaspoons olive oil

1 cup cherry tomatoes, halved

1 medium green bell pepper, diced

1 medium red bell pepper, diced

1 medium yellow onion, chopped fine

1 can *(14 ounces)* cannellini beans, drained

1 can *(13.75 ounces)* artichoke hearts, in water, drained and sliced

1 tablespoon sacha inchi oil *(or olive oil)*

Salt, pepper, and dried basil

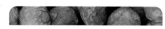

The omega-3s from sacha inchi oil can help prevent blood from clogging by keeping saturated fats mobile in the bloodstream. They also help with the fluidity of cellular membranes so that oxygen can flow from red blood cells to the body's tissues.

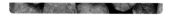

Per Serving: Kcal 205, Protein 9g, Carb 36g, Fat 5g, Sodium 301.5mg, Dietary Fiber 7.5g
Daily Values: Fiber 31%, Vit C 122%, Vit A 27%, Vit D 5 0%, Calcium 10%, Iron 13%

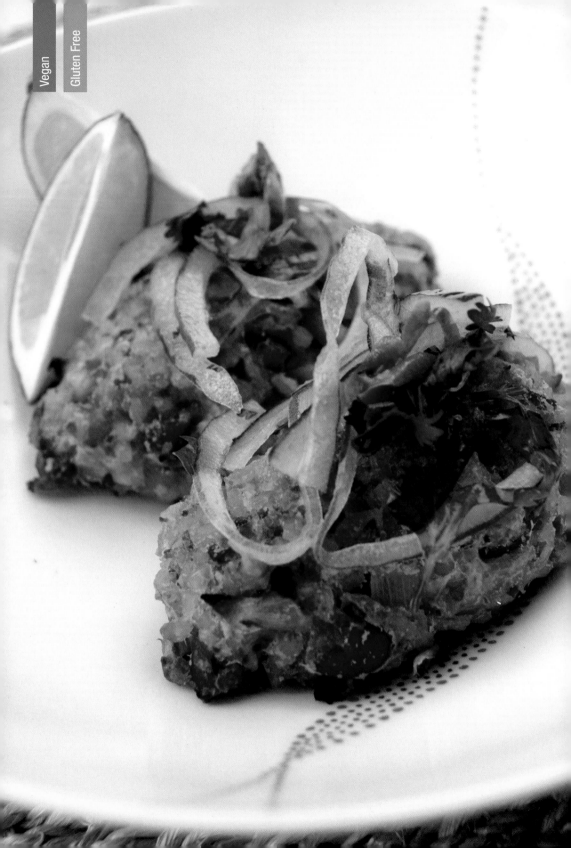

TACU TACU

Tacu Tacu is the combination of leftover rice and beans where the food is deep-fried. Traditionally, the dish is eaten with eggs at breakfast. We infused the classic fare by baking instead of frying for a light and healthful version. Try eating this with any of your favorite proteins of choice at any meal your heart desires.

1 tablespoon canola oil

1 large yellow onion, chopped fine

3 cloves garlic, crushed

1 tablespoon ají amarillo paste (*or mild chili paste*)

1½ cups cooked pinto beans

2 cups cooked brown rice

Oil spray

❶ Heat the oil in a large sauté pan over medium heat. Add the onion and garlic and cook for 3 to 5 minutes or until soft.

❷ Add the ají and beans and gently mash them into the onion mixture using your spatula or a fork. Add the rice and continue cooking until a dense mass forms. Turn off the heat and let cool.

❸ Preheat the oven to 400 degrees F. Lightly oil a baking sheet.

❹ Divide the tacu tacu into eight equal portions. Gently roll each portion with your hands to form a 2 × 3–inch oval and place them on the baking sheet. Once all of the ovals are formed and placed on the pan, coat the tops with a light layer of oil spray and bake until crisp and golden, for 20 to 30 minutes. Eat warm.

Beans are a good source of fiber. Increased fiber intake benefits a number of gastrointestinal disorders, including acid reflux disease, constipation, diverticulitis, duodenal ulcer, and hemorrhoids.

Per Serving: Kcal 125, Protein 4.5g, Carb 21.5g, Fat 2.5g, Sodium 38.5mg, Dietary Fiber 4g
Daily Values: Fiber 16%, Vit C 3%, Vit A 0%, Vit D 5 0%, Calcium 2%, Iron 5%

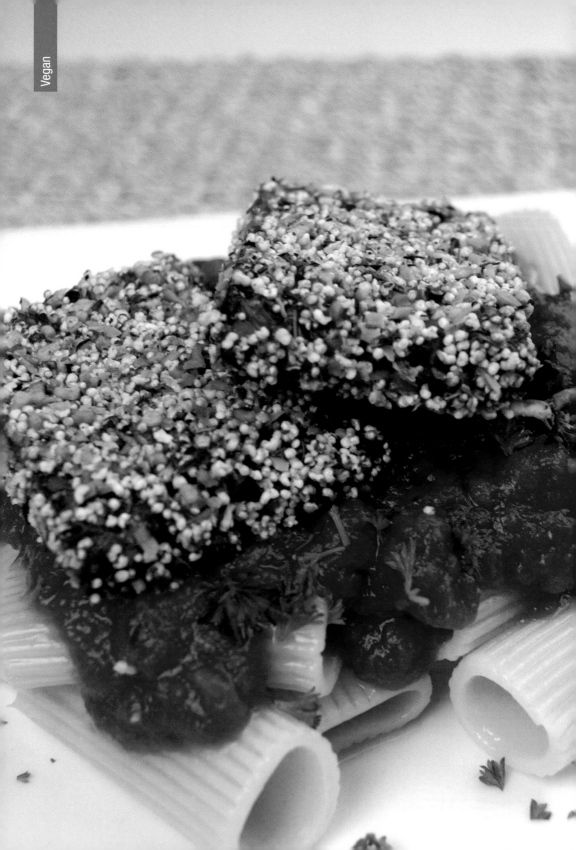

TEMPEH MILANESE

Servings: 8 ♦ Serving size: 1 ounce

Looking for an Italian-fusion recipe? This is a must-try dish, and it's gluten-free. Instead of using bread crumbs, we use popped kiwicha to increase the nutrition profile while adding a hearty crunch.

1 block *(8 ounces)* **tempeh**

½ cup milk

1 tablespoon olive oil

Juice of ½ lemon *(about 1½ teaspoons)*

4 cloves garlic, crushed

Salt and pepper

½ cup popped kiwicha *(see recipe on page 220)*

¼ cup grated Parmesan cheese

½ teaspoon salt

½ teaspoon dried thyme

½ teaspoon dried oregano

½ teaspoon dried marjoram

Oil spray

❶ Cut the tempeh into four equal-size rectangles. Cut them again until you have a total of eight equal-size rectangles. Carefully slice each rectangle so that it is half its original thickness. Place the tempeh slices in a casserole dish to form a single layer.

❷ Combine the milk, oil, lemon juice, and garlic in a small bowl. Season with salt and pepper to taste. Pour the marinade over the tempeh to cover, and let it marinate at room temperature for an hour or overnight in the refrigerator.

❸ To make the "breading," combine the kiwicha, Parmesan cheese, salt, thyme, oregano, and marjoram in a small bowl. Set aside.

❹ Preheat the oven to 400 degrees F. Lightly spray a baking sheet with the oil spray.

❺ Dip the tempeh slices in the kiwicha breading to form an even layer over the surface. Place the slices on the baking sheet.

❻ Bake the tempeh for 15 to 20 minutes, flipping halfway through the baking process, until crisp and golden.

NOTE: Tempeh Milanese is best if eaten on the day it's prepared.

With a balanced carbohydrate and protein content and no gluten, kiwicha is perfect for people with celiac disease, gluten sensitivity, and intolerance.

Per Serving: Kcal 102, Protein 7g, Carb 6g, Fat 6g, Sodium 339mg, Dietary Fiber 0.5g
Daily Values: Fiber 2%, Vit C 3%, Vit A 1%, Vit D 5 2%, Calcium 9%, Iron 7%

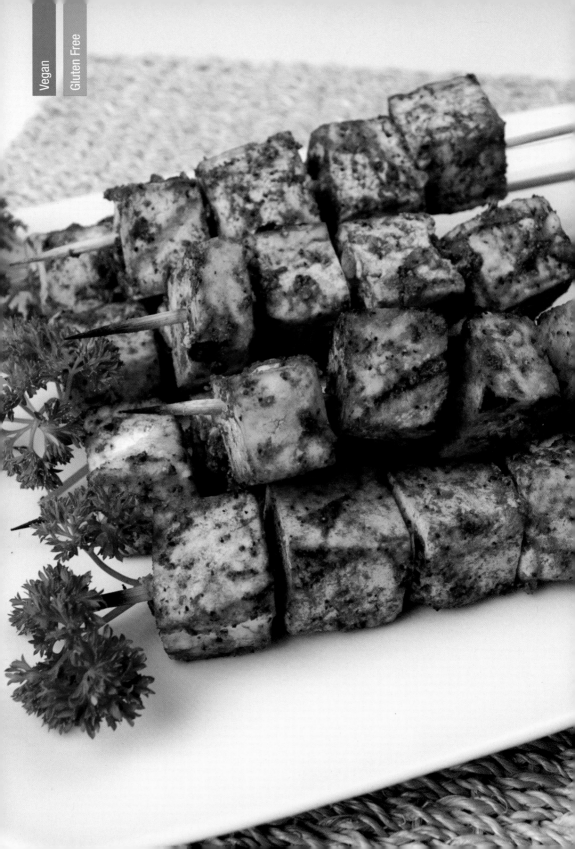

TOFU À LA PANCA

Servings: 8 ♦ Serving size: 1 skewer

Peru has a famous street food called "anticuchos." Anticuchos are generally made with meat skewered on sticks. We've provided you with a vegan version of the classic street food while maintaining all the delicious flavors, so you instantly get transported to the marvelous streets of Peru.

12 cloves garlic, crushed

1 tablespoon ground cumin

¼ cup ají panca paste *(or mild chili paste)*

¼ cup white wine vinegar

1 teaspoon salt

1 tablespoon pepper

1 tablespoon canola oil

2 blocks *(14 ounces each)* firm tofu, cut into 1½-inch pieces

8 wooden skewers

❶ Place the wooden skewers in a casserole dish and fill with water to cover. Let them soak for 30 to 60 minutes before using.

❷ Combine the garlic, cumin, ají, vinegar, salt, pepper, and oil in a large, shallow bowl. Mix with a fork to create a smooth, homogeneous mixture. Add the tofu to the marinade and toss to coat. Let it marinate for 60 minutes at room temperature or overnight in the refrigerator.

❸ Divide the tofu among the skewers, making sure they have lots of sauce on them.

❹ Heat up your grill according to the manufacturer's instructions. Grill the skewers, turning them as necessary until a light char forms. Remove and eat warm.

Per Serving: Kcal 121, Protein 9.5g, Carb 5.5g, Fat 5.5g, Sodium 434mg, Dietary Fiber 1g
Daily Values: Fiber 5%, Vit C 3%, Vit A 0%, Vit D 5 0%, Calcium 15%, Iron 9%

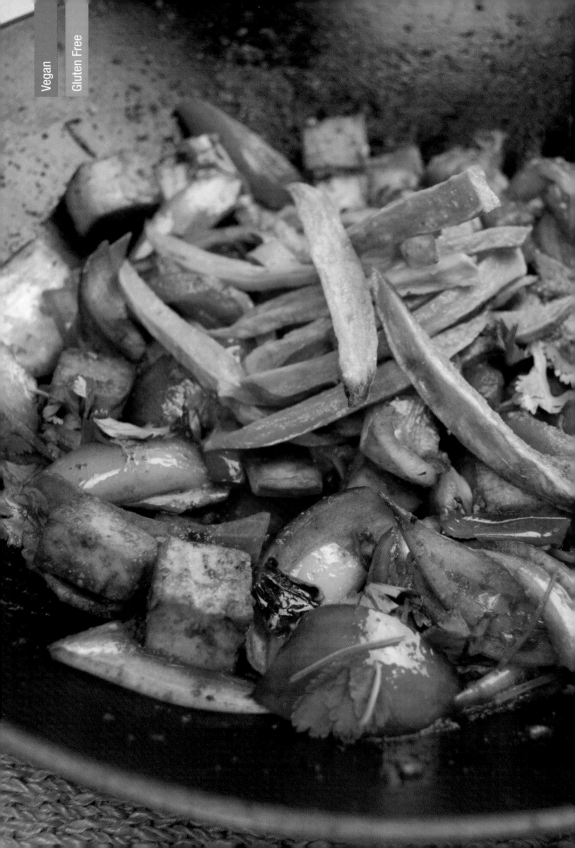

TOFU SALTADO

Lomo saltado is a popular dish in Peru. It is a unique dish in that it carries an Asian influence, common to dishes found in the ubiquitous Chifa (Peruvian Chinese) restaurants, as well as in many home kitchens. While lomo saltado is traditionally prepared using beef tri-tip, we made a vegan version using tofu.

28 ounces (2 blocks) extra firm, lite tofu

3 tablespoons low-sodium soy sauce

2 teaspoons ground cumin

1 tablespoon canola oil

2 medium red onions, coarsely chopped

1 clove garlic, minced

1 tablespoon ají amarillo paste (or mild chili paste)

2 tablespoons balsamic vinegar

2 large tomatoes, coarsely chopped

Handful of fresh cilantro

❶ Cut the tofu into 1-inch cubes and put in a large, shallow bowl. Cover the tofu with the soy sauce and cumin, and let it marinate at room temperature for 1 hour.

❷ Put the oil in a large sauté pan or wok over medium-high heat. Drain the tofu, reserving the marinade. Add the tofu to the pan and cook until nicely browned.

❸ Add the onions, garlic, ají, vinegar, and leftover marinade to the pan. Cook for 2 to 3 minutes and then turn off the heat. Add the tomato and cilantro to the pan and stir to combine.

NOTE: Tofu saltado will keep in the refrigerator for three to five days.

Per Serving: Kcal 236.5, Protein 23.5g, Carb 12.5g, Fat 13.5g, Sodium 584.5mg, Dietary Fiber 1.5g
Daily Values: Fiber 6%, Vit C 13%, Vit A 9%, Vit D 5 0%, Calcium 12%, Iron 26%

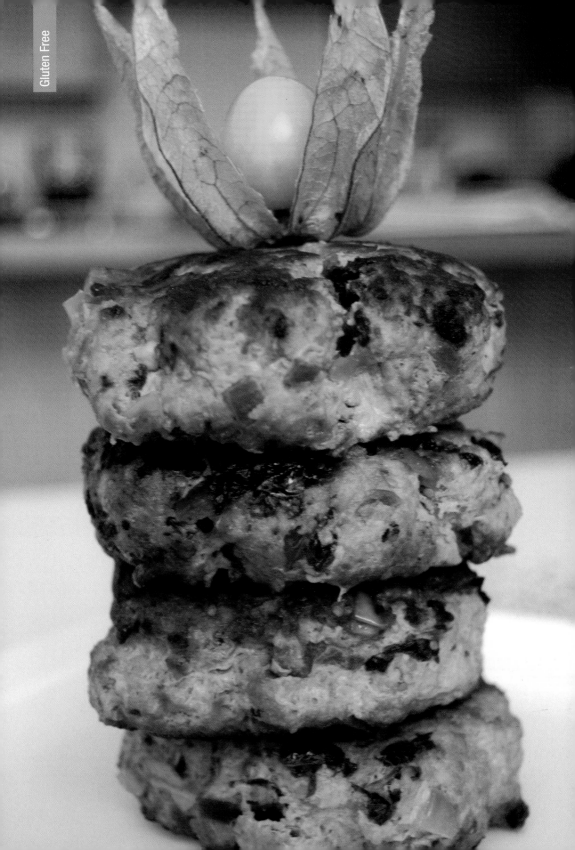

TURKEY PICHUBERRY BURGER PATTIES

Servings: 5 ◆ Serving size: 1 patty

Tired of your bland, boring turkey burgers?
Liven them up with an explosion of flavor from
the cilantro and pichuberries. You'll astonish your
taste buds and do the happy dance after eating
these burgers!

1 tablespoon canola oil

½ medium red onion, minced

½ cup pichuberry halves

½ cup chopped cilantro

1 pound 4 ounces lean ground turkey

Salt and pepper

Oil spray

❶ Heat the oil in a large saucepan over medium heat. When the oil is hot, add the onion and sauté until soft and fragrant, for about 5 minutes. Stir in the pichuberries and cilantro and cook for another few minutes until tender. Let the vegetables cool completely before moving on to the next step.

❷ Combine the sautéed vegetables with the ground turkey in a medium bowl. Season with salt and pepper to taste.

❸ Divide the turkey mixture into five equal portions, forming each into a 4-inch patty.

❹ Heat a large sauté pan over medium heat. Lightly spray the pan with oil and panfry each burger patty for 5 minutes on each side or to desired doneness.

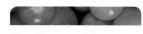

The oil extracted from the skin and pulp of the pichuberry contains high levels of plant sterols. Plant sterols are known to help reduce cholesterol levels, especially bad cholesterol (LDL).

Per Serving: Kcal 212, Protein 20g, Carb 3.5g, Fat 12.5g, Sodium 579.5mg, Dietary Fiber 0.5g
Daily Values: Fiber 2%, Vit C 4%, Vit A 7%, Vit D 5 5%, Calcium 2%, Iron 9%

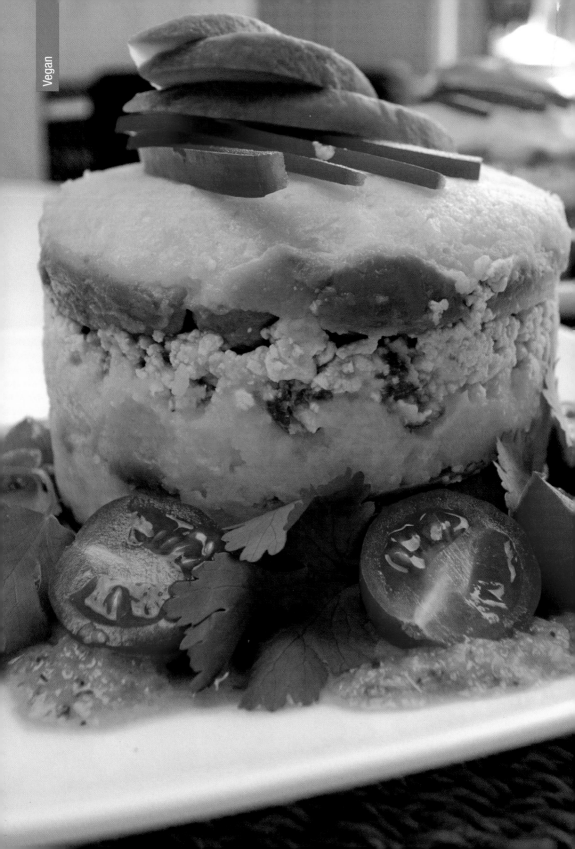

VEGGIE CAUSA WITH TOFU

Servings: 4 ♦ Serving size: ½ of one causa

"Causa" is a Peruvian dish consisting of mashed potatoes with a filling of your choice. Here we filled the potatoes with tofu and avocado.

❶ Put the potatoes in a medium saucepan with enough water to cover by 1 inch. Bring to a boil over medium-high heat and let them cook until tender, for 20 to 30 minutes. When the potatoes are done, drain and let cool. Mash the potatoes using a potato ricer or masher, then put them in a medium bowl and set aside.

❷ Add the lime juice, 3 tablespoons of the ají, and the oil to the potatoes. Season with salt and pepper to taste. Mix thoroughly to evenly distribute the ají. Set aside.

❸ Coat a large sauté pan with cooking spray and place over medium heat. Add the tofu to the pan. Before the pan gets too hot, mash the tofu with a potato masher or fork to resemble small curds. Add the remaining ají paste to the pan, along with salt and pepper to taste. Cook the tofu until lightly browned, making sure not to dry it out too much. Set aside to cool.

❹ Oil the inside of the metal rings (or causa molds) and place them on a sheet pan or a large plate lined with parchment paper.

❺ To prepare the causas, divide the potato mixture into six portions, the avocado into four portions, and the tofu into four portions. Place one portion of the mashed potatoes into each of the two rings and press down to form an even layer. Add a layer of avocado followed by a layer of tofu. Repeat layering, ending with a final layer of potato.

❻ Make sure the layers are pressed down firmly, then remove the molds. Serve with the Ají Vinaigrette.

3 medium yellow potatoes, peeled and cut into 1-inch cubes

¼ cup key lime juice *(or lime juice)*

5 tablespoons ají amarillo paste *(or mild chili paste)*

2 tablespoons canola oil

Oil spray

Salt and pepper

14 ounces *(1 package)* medium tofu, cubed

1 avocado, thinly sliced

1 recipe Ají Vinaigrette *(see recipe on page 240)*

2 metal rings, about 4 inches in diameter by 3 inches tall *(or use causa molds)*

Per Serving: Kcal 319, Protein 12g, Carb 21.5g, Fat 21.5g, Sodium 518mg, Dietary Fiber 4g
Daily Values: Fiber 16%, Vit C 25%, Vit A 1%, Vit D 5 0%, Calcium 14%, Iron 18%

WEEKEND OREGANO ROASTED CHICKEN

Servings: 6 ♦ Serving Size: 4 ounces

1½ pounds skinless chicken breasts

Juice of 1 lemon *(about 3 tablespoons)*

1 tablespoon olive oil

¼ cup dry oregano

Salt and pepper

Make this recipe on a Sunday so you have chicken to use whenever you need it throughout the following week. You can use this chicken in multiple recipes from the book. It can be added to salads, soups, grain dishes, and more.

❶ Preheat the oven to 450 degrees F.

❷ Place the chicken breasts in a roasting pan. Pour the juice and oil over the breasts and toss them to coat. Sprinkle the chicken breasts with the oregano and salt and pepper to taste.

❸ Bake the chicken for 22 minutes or until crisp and golden on the outside and moist on the inside. Remove it from the oven and let it cool for 5 to 10 minutes before slicing.

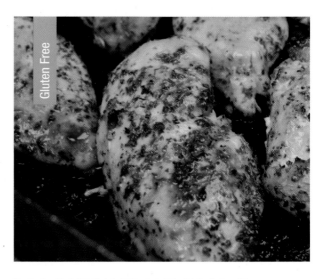

Gluten Free

Per Serving: Kcal 156, Protein 26.5g, Carb 2.5g, Fat 4g, Sodium 74mg, Dietary Fiber 1.5g
Daily Values: Fiber 5%, Vit C 11%, Vit A 5%, Vit D 5 0%, Calcium 6%, Iron 12%

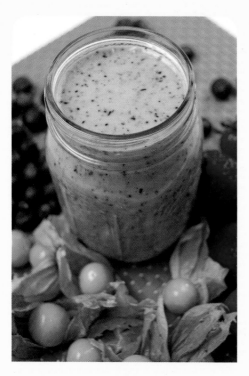

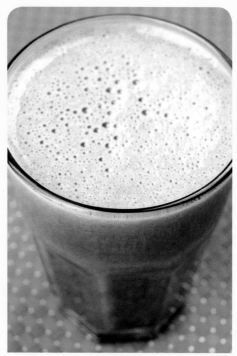

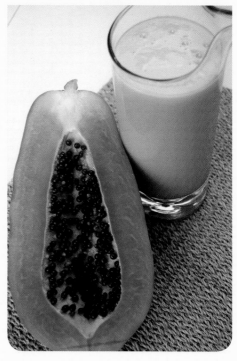

Shakes,
Smoothies
& Elixirs

CHIA CACAO PROTEIN SHAKE

Servings: 1 ◆ Serving size: 3 cups

2 cups unsweetened almond milk

1 small banana

2 tablespoons cacao powder

1 tablespoon chia seeds

1 scoop *(20 to 25 grams)* protein powder *(rice, pea, or whey)*

Start your day right with this fast, protein-packed, antioxidant-filled superhero shake.

❶ Put all the ingredients in a blender and process until smooth. Add water, if needed, to reach desired consistency.

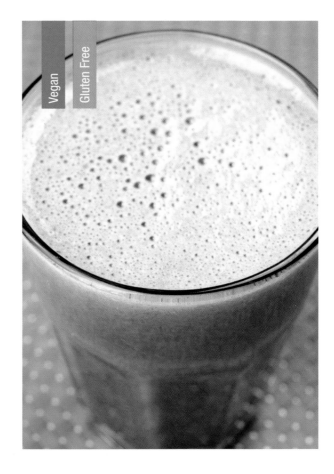

Vegan

Gluten Free

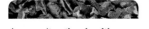

Among its other health benefits, cacao is a natural appetite suppressant, so it can help reduce food cravings and aid in weight loss.

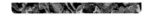

Per Serving: Kcal 372, Protein 31g, Carb 43.5g, Fat 10g, Sodium 383mg, Dietary Fiber 10g
Daily Values: Fiber 40%, Vit C 20%, Vit A 22%, Vit D 5 50%, Calcium 13%, Iron 33%

SILKY PAPAYA SMOOTHIE

Servings: 1 ◆ Serving size: 4 cups

Delight in a quick and easy breakfast blast of flavor.

❶ Put the papaya, tofu, and yogurt into a blender and process until smooth, adding water, if needed, to reach the desired consistency. The smoothie will keep in the refrigerator for one to three days.

2 cups cubed papaya

8 ounces (*½ block*) silken tofu

¾ cup low-fat coconut yogurt

¼ to ¾ cup water

Vegan

Gluten Free

The fiber in papaya can bind to cancer-causing toxins and flush them away from healthy cells, thus helping to prevent colon cancer. In addition, papaya's beta-carotene, folate, and vitamins C and E are also linked to a reduced risk of colon cancer. Those with increased risk of colon cancer should increase their intake of papaya.

Per Serving: Kcal 351.5, Protein 12.5g, Carb 46g, Fat 12.5g, Sodium 37mg, Dietary Fiber 8g
Daily Values: Fiber 32%, Vit C 288%, Vit A 61%, Vit D 5 0%, Calcium 42%, Iron 18%

TRIPLE-BERRY BREAKFAST SMOOTHIE

Servings: 1 ♦ Serving size: 2½ cups

½ cup pichuberries

½ cup sliced strawberries

½ cup blueberries

1 cup plain, nonfat kefir

1 scoop *(16 grams)* protein powder *(rice, pea, or whey)*

Ramp up your antioxidants with this powerhouse shake full of probiotics and a complete protein. Get ready to increase your metabolism and burn the belly fat.

❶ Put all the ingredients in a blender and process until smooth. Add water, if needed, to reach the desired consistency.

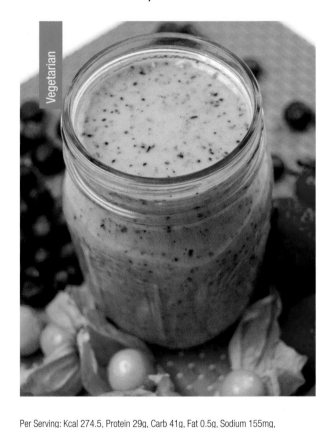

Vegetarian

Pichuberries contain a large group of naturally occurring active chemical compounds called withanolides. There has been a strong link between withanolides and the inhibition of cancer cell growth.

Per Serving: Kcal 274.5, Protein 29g, Carb 41g, Fat 0.5g, Sodium 155mg, Dietary Fiber 7g
Daily Values: Fiber 27%, Vit C 98%, Vit A 36%, Vit D 5 51%, Calcium 32%, Iron 13%

YOUTHH2O GREEN MACHINE

Servings: 1 ◆ Serving size: 3½ cups

Jump-start the antiaging process and utilize the youthH2O age-defying system with Peruvian power foods: maca, camu camu, and purple corn extracts. Drink this smoothie to stimulate, replenish, and reactivate your body to fight signs of aging and boost energy.

1½ cups coconut water

1 cup cubed papaya

2 cups spinach

¼ cup chopped parsley

1 shot *(2 ounces)* youthH2O

❶ Put all the ingredients in a blender and puree until smooth. Add water until it's the desired consistency. Drink immediately.

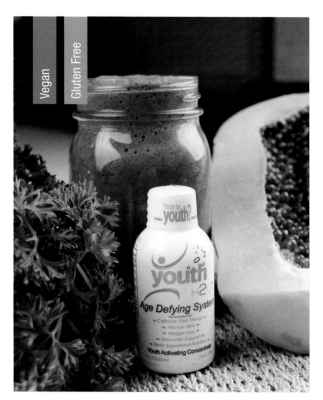

The camu berry is one of the world's most potent sources of vitamin C— packing more than sixty times the amount per serving than the almighty orange. Synthetic vitamin C does not produce collagen. However, vitamin C from camu camu is in its natural form, and natural vitamin C has been shown to repair and produce collagen.

Per Serving: Kcal 157.5, Protein 4.5g, Carb 3.5g, Fat 0.5g, Sodium 168.5mg, Dietary Fiber 17g
Daily Values: Fiber 17%, Vit C 716%, Vit A 169%, Vit D 5 0%, Calcium 18%, Iron 15%

YOUTHH2O TROPICAL INCAN EXPLOSION

Servings: 1 ◆ Serving size: 3½ cups

1 cup coconut water

½ cup diced yellow tomato

½ cup cubed pineapple

1 cup pichuberries

1 teaspoon ground turmeric

1 shot *(2 ounces)* youthH2O

We used a shot of youthH2O to provide you with a powerhouse of phytonutrients and give you energy and detoxification. Begin your day with an explosion of antioxidant health.

❶ Put all the ingredients in a blender and puree until smooth. Add water until it's the desired consistency. Drink immediately.

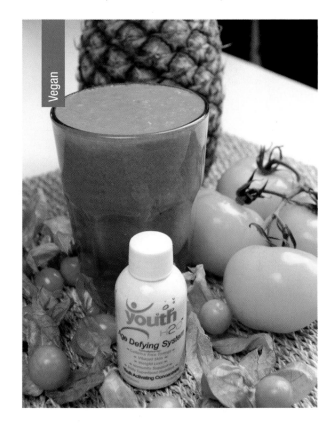

Vegan

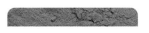

Maca, one of the Peruvian superfoods in youthH2O, is rich in amino acids. Amino acids are the building blocks of our DNA. YouthH2O contains nearly all of the essential amino acids.

Per Serving: Kcal 205.5, Protein 5g, Carb 46g, Fat 1g, Sodium 156.5mg, Dietary Fiber 3.5g
Daily Values: Fiber 13%, Vit C 607%, Vit A 50%, Vit D 5 52%, Calcium 8%, Iron 8%

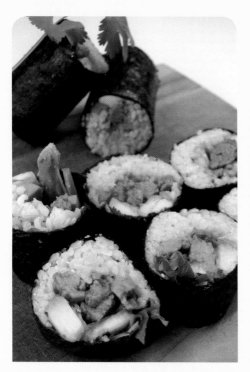
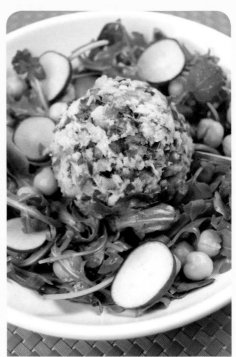
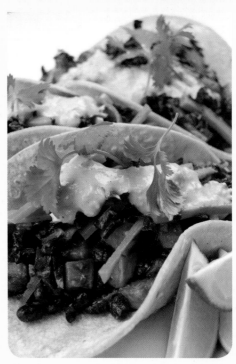

Salads,
Sandwiches
& Wraps

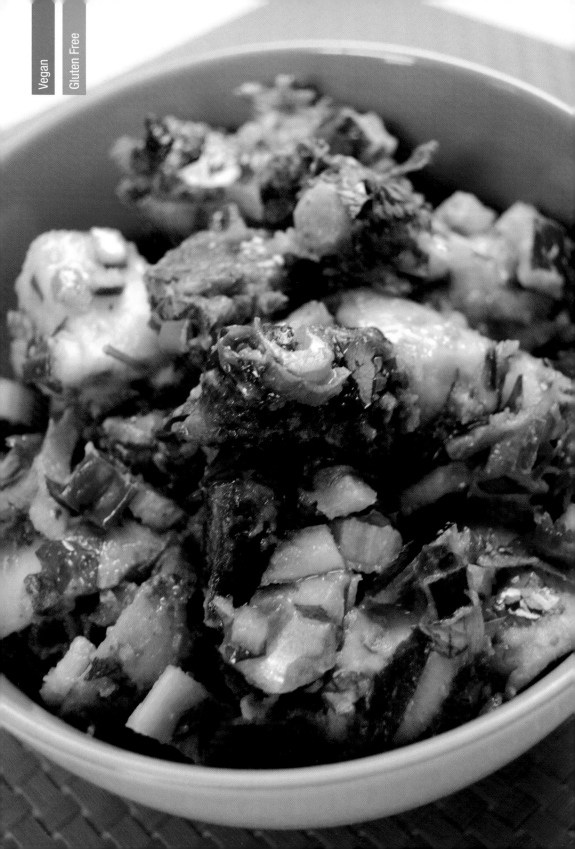

ANDEAN POTATO SALAD

Servings: 6 ♦ Serving size: 1⅔ cups

Relish the benefits of using two different kinds of potatoes in this lip-smacking salad—perfect for a picnic.

❶ Wash the potatoes and put them in a large stockpot. Add enough water to the pot so that the potatoes are submerged under 2 inches of water. Bring the water to a boil and cook the potatoes until tender. The potatoes are done when each can be easily pierced with a sharp knife. Pour the potatoes into a colander and let them cool completely before mixing with the remaining ingredients.

❷ Put the shallot and garlic in a small bowl. Add the white vinegar and mix to combine. Set aside.

❸ Put the celery, scallions, parsley, cilantro, oil, mustard, and ají in a large mixing bowl. Toss to combine.

❹ Once the potatoes are completely cool, cut them into 1-inch chunks and add them to the large mixing bowl along with the vinegar mixture. Toss to combine. Season with salt and pepper to taste. Refrigerate for 1 hour before serving.

1 pound purple potatoes

1 pound yellow potatoes

1 shallot, minced

2 cloves garlic, crushed

3 tablespoons white wine vinegar

4 medium stalks celery, thinly sliced

4 green scallions, thinly sliced

½ cup chopped flat-leaf parsley

½ cup chopped cilantro

¼ cup sacha inchi oil *(or olive oil)*

2 tablespoons mustard

2 tablespoons ají amarillo paste *(or mild chili paste)*

Salt and pepper

Anthocyanins from purple potatoes can help control blood sugar levels by breaking up glucose.

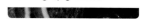

Per Serving: Kcal 239, Protein 4g, Carb 33g, Fat 10g, Sodium 184.5mg, Dietary Fiber 2.5g
Daily Values: Fiber 10%, Vit C 39%, Vit A 6%, Vit D 5 0%, Calcium 4%, Iron 13%

AVOCADO QUESO FRESCO SANDWICH

Serves: 1 ♦ Serving size: 1 sandwich

2 slices whole-grain bread

½ medium avocado, sliced

3 ounces low-fat queso fresco, sliced

¼ cup basil leaves

In Peru there is a classic sandwich called "triple" with eggs, avocado, and tomato. This is a twist on the classic Peruvian delight. You will love every bite.

❶ Toast the bread, if you prefer. Layer the avocado slices, queso fresco, and basil between the slices of toast. Enjoy!

NOTE: If you would like to pack this sandwich for lunch to eat later in the day, use untoasted bread and squeeze a little lime juice on the avocado to keep it from browning.

Eating avocados can help decrease blood triglycerides and increase HDL (the "good" cholesterol). Both short- and long-term studies show that eating avocados also decreases high blood pressure, which lowers the risk of developing cardiovascular disease.

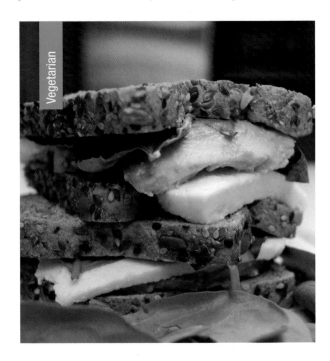

Vegetarian

Per Serving: Kcal 477, Protein 19g, Carb 54g, Fat 23g, Sodium 708mg, Dietary Fiber 11g
Daily Values: Fiber 43%, Vit C 13%, Vit A 21%, Vit D 5 0%, Calcium 32%, Iron 19%

BEET & ORANGE SALAD WITH PICHUBERRY CHAMPAGNE VINAIGRETTE

Servings: 4 ♦ Serving size: 1½ cups

The earthy flavor of the sacha inchi oil balances the sweetness from the oranges. The explosion of color from the red beets and oranges will wow your taste buds—a perfect summer dish.

4 large beets, stemmed and peeled

2 large oranges, peeled

1 recipe Champagne Vinaigrette with Pichuberries *(see recipe on page 243)*

❶ Put the beets in a medium stockpot and fill with enough water to cover. Bring to a boil over medium heat, cover, then reduce to a simmer for 30 to 40 minutes or until the beets are tender when pierced with a fork. Drain the beets and let them cool to room temperature.

❷ Slice the cooled beets and oranges into ½-inch rounds. Arrange the slices on a plate by alternating the beets with the oranges.

❸ Drizzle the salad with the vinaigrette dressing right before serving.

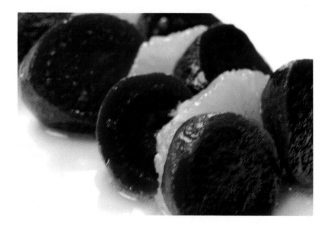

Per Serving: Kcal 93.5, Protein 2g, Carb 18.5g, Fat 2g, Sodium 67mg, Dietary Fiber 4g
Daily Values: Fiber 16%, Vit C 77%, Vit A 5%, Vit D 5 2%, Calcium 4%, Iron 4%

BLACK BEAN & SWEET POTATO THAI FUSION TACOS

Servings: 10 ♦ Serving size: 1 taco

Vegan

Gluten Free

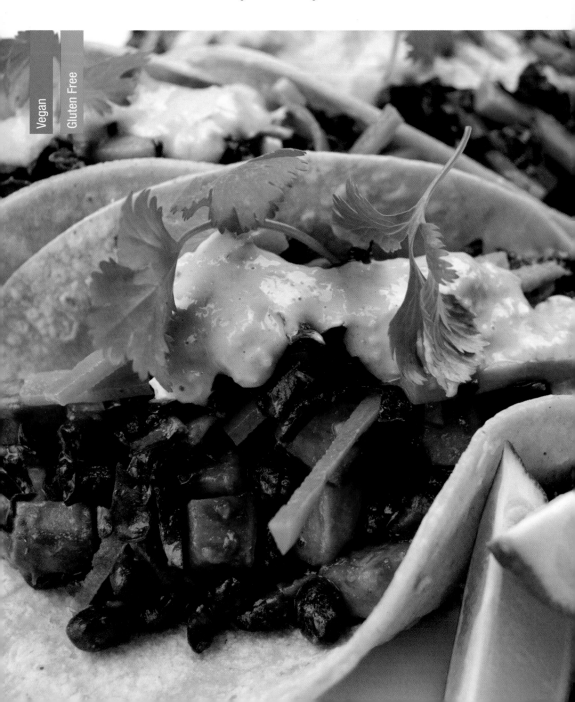

Jamie Farnsworth is a food blogger with a vegan website: Girl Eats Greens (girleatsgreens.com). She naturally fuses recipes, just like us.

TO MAKE THE FILLING:

❶ Spray a medium-size skillet with the oil spray and place it over medium heat. Add the sweet potatoes and sauté until they start to brown a bit.

❷ Add half of the garlic and the black beans until the beans are heated through and the garlic has cooked.

❸ Add ¼ cup of the coconut milk, the cayenne, and the cumin and mix well.

❹ Reduce the heat to low to keep the filling warm, if you're not quite ready to serve yet. This will also give the flavors a chance to meld.

TO MAKE THE CARROT AND KALE SLAW:

Put the kale and carrots in a large bowl. Add 1 tablespoon of the lime juice and ½ teaspoon of the sesame oil to the bowl. Toss until the kale and carrots are evenly coated.

TO MAKE THE PEANUT SAUCE:

Cut the jalapeño in half and remove the seeds. Put the peanut butter, jalapeño, water, and the remaining coconut milk, garlic, lime juice, and sesame oil in the bowl of a food processor. Pulse until the jalapeño and garlic are chopped up and everything is well incorporated.

TO ASSEMBLE:

Warm up the tortillas in the oven at 350 degrees F or toast them a bit by placing them in a pan over high heat for about 10 seconds on each side (my favorite method). Put the sweet potato and black bean mixture on a tortilla, followed by the slaw and peanut sauce. Garnish with a few bits of cilantro. Serve with a slice of lime and enjoy!

Olive oil spray

1 medium sweet potato, chopped *(about 1½ cups)*

2 cloves garlic, minced

1 can *(15 ounces)* black beans, rinsed and drained

¼ cup plus 2 tablespoons low-fat coconut milk

¼ teaspoon cayenne pepper

1 teaspoon cumin

1 cup shredded kale

1 cup julienned carrots *(about half of a large carrot)*

Juice of 1 medium lime *(about 2 tablespoons)*

1½ teaspoons sesame oil

1 jalapeño

¼ cup peanut butter

1 tablespoon water

10 small corn tortillas

Cilantro and extra lime slices for garnish *(optional)*

Per Serving: Kcal 151, Protein 5.5g, Carb 23.5g, Fat 5.5g, Sodium 217.5mg, Dietary Fiber 5g
Daily Values: Fiber 20%, Vit C 20%, Vit A 68%, Vit D 5 0%, Calcium 6%, Iron 7%

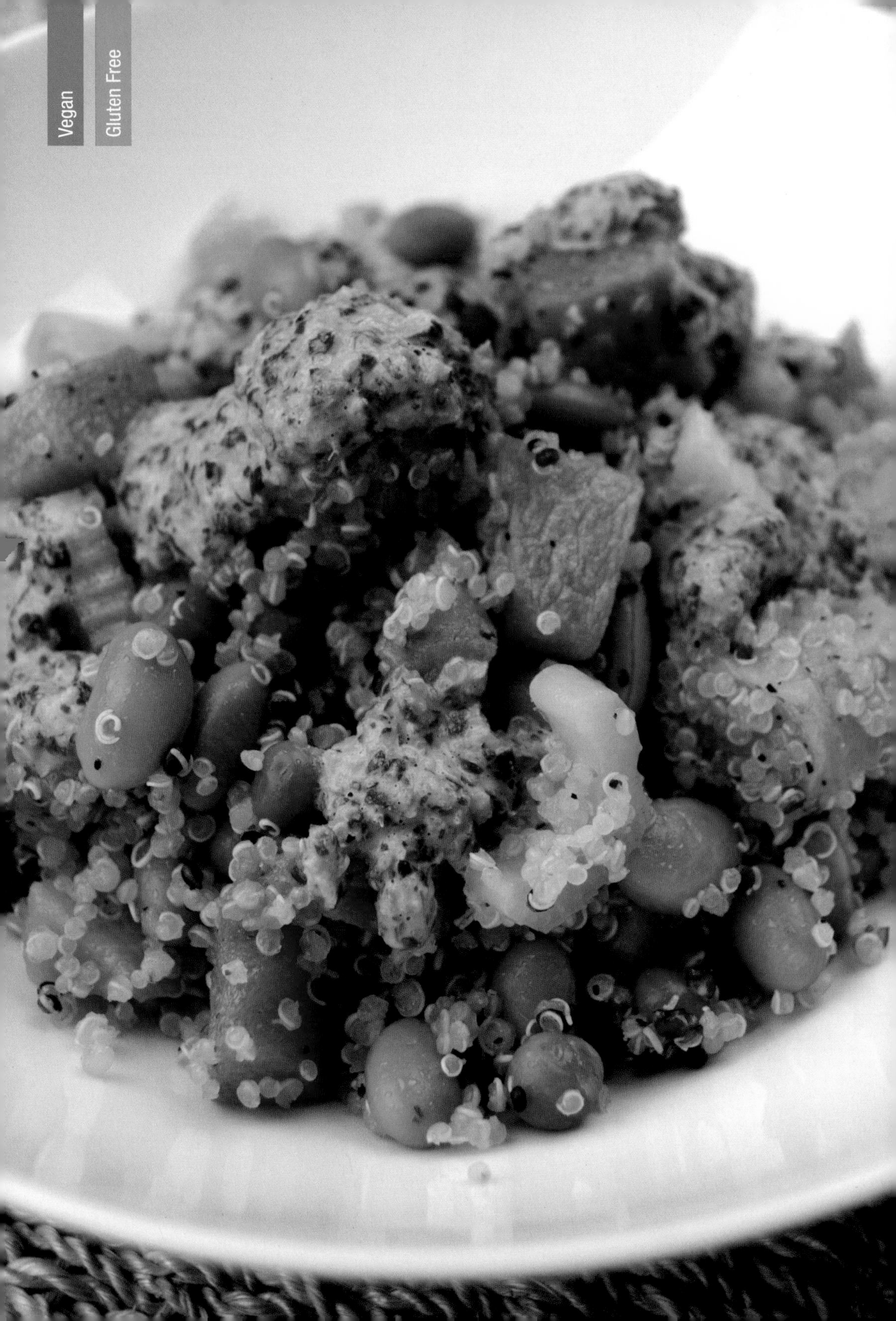
Vegan
Gluten Free

BUTTERNUT SQUASH & LEGUMES QUINOA SALAD

Servings: 10 ♦ Serving size: 1 cup

Bursting with flavor, this hearty salad is a complete meal in one—full of proteins, carbs, and fats.

❶ Preheat the oven to 400 degrees F. Lightly spray a small baking sheet with the oil spray.

❷ Place the squash on the baking sheet. Lightly spray it with the oil spray and season with salt and pepper. Bake for 30 to 40 minutes until lightly browned and tender. Set aside to cool.

❸ Bring a medium-size pot of water to a boil over high heat. Add the edamame and peas and cook until tender, for about 5 minutes. Drain and let cool.

❹ Combine the quinoa, celery, and oil in a large bowl. Add the cooled squash, edamame, and peas to the bowl and toss to combine. Season with salt and pepper.

Olive oil spray

4 cups diced butternut squash *(about 1 pound 4 ounces)*

Salt and pepper

2 cups shelled edamame, fresh or frozen

1 cup shelled peas, fresh or frozen

2 cups cooked quinoa *(see recipe on page 238)*

1 large celery rib, sliced

2 tablespoons olive oil

Quinoa contains phytosterols, which have been linked to preventing oxidative damage, preventing cancer growth, and lowering cholesterol.

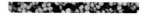

Per Serving: Kcal 133, Protein 5.5g, Carb 19g, Fat 5g, Sodium 258mg, Dietary Fiber 3.7g
Daily Values: Fiber 15%, Vit C 28%, Vit A 95%, Vit D 5 0%, Calcium 5%, Iron 10%

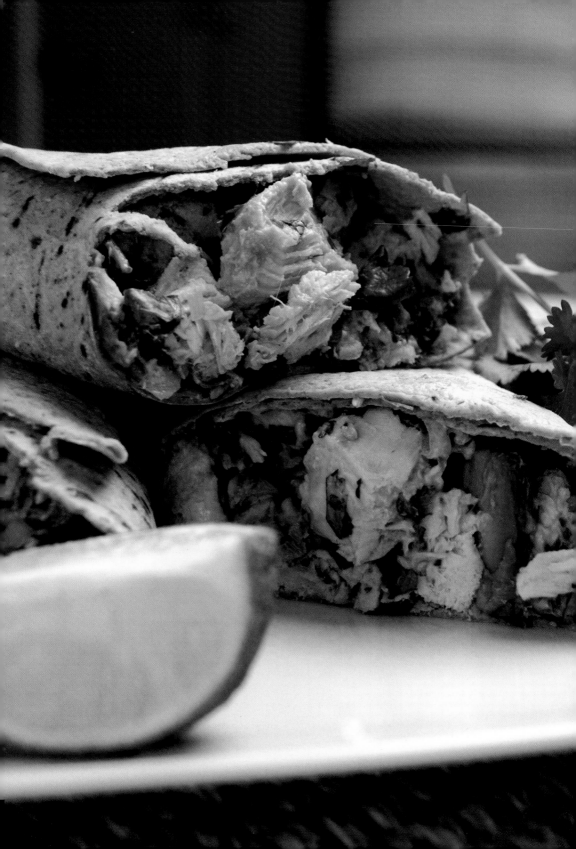

CHICKEN AVOCADO WRAP

Servings: 4 ◆ Serving size: ½ wrap

You'll relish this Mediterranean-infused dish with classic Peruvian flavors from cilantro and lime. This classic roasted chicken recipe can be found throughout Peru and is very common cuisine.

❶ Put the chicken, avocado, scallions, cilantro, yogurt, and lime juice in a medium bowl and toss to combine. Season with salt and pepper to taste.

❷ Divide the mixture among two flatbreads and tightly roll each into a wrap. Cut each wrap into two halves before serving. Eat these the day you prepare them.

2 cups shredded Weekend Oregano Roasted Chicken *(see recipe on page 152)*

1 avocado, peeled, pitted, and cubed

2 green scallions, finely chopped

½ cup chopped cilantro

2 tablespoons low-fat Greek yogurt

Juice of 1 lime *(about 1½ to 2 tablespoons)*

Salt and pepper

2 whole wheat flatbreads, tortillas, or lavash

Per Serving: Kcal 234.5, Protein 18g, Carb 19.5g, Fat 11g, Sodium 295mg, Dietary Fiber 6g
Daily Values: Fiber 23%, Vit C 18%, Vit A 8%, Vit D 5 0%, Calcium 6%, Iron 11%

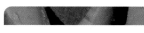

Many studies show that a diet rich in avocados and its many phytochemicals may help to prevent cancer.

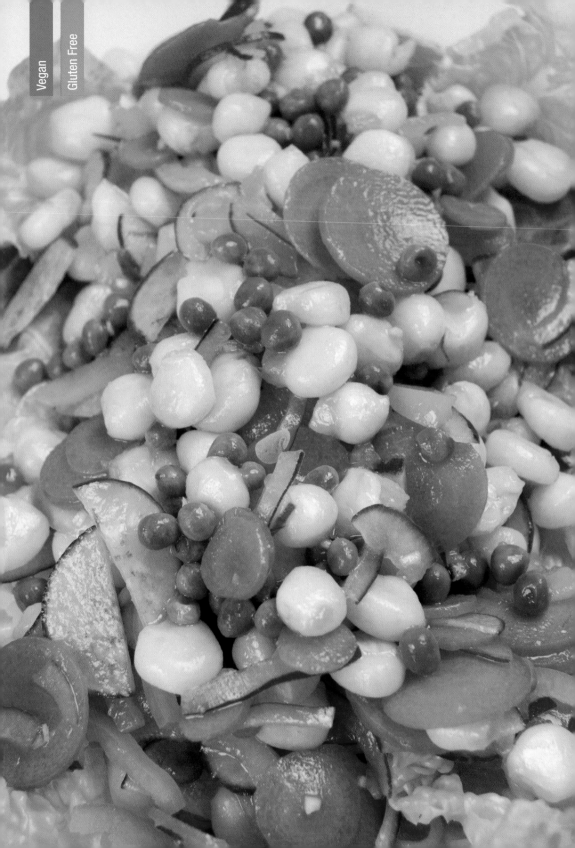

CHOCLO CHOPPED SALAD

Servings: 5 ♦ Serving size: 1 cup

Our colleague and chef, Chenoa Bol, shared this delectable recipe with us where she marries the sweetness of choclo, an oversized corn kernel from the Andes, with the fresh garden crunch of thinly sliced raw vegetables. It's a colorful salad that is pleasing to the eyes and the appetite.

❶ Put the garlic, onion, vinegar, and lime juice in a small bowl. Mix and set aside to marinate for 15 minutes.

❷ Combine the choclo, bell pepper, carrot, ají, and oil in a large bowl. Add the marinated onion mixture and toss to combine. Season with salt to taste.

1 clove garlic, minced

¼ medium red onion, cut into half-moon slivers

2 tablespoons white wine vinegar

1 tablespoon lime juice

1 pound cooked choclo *(see recipe on page 235)*

½ medium yellow bell pepper, cut into matchsticks

1 medium carrot, sliced into thin rounds

2 tablespoons ají amarillo paste *(or mild chili paste)*

1 tablespoon sacha inchi oil *(or olive oil)*

Salt

Per Serving: Kcal 170, Protein 4g, Carb 34g, Fat 3g, Sodium 130.5mg, Dietary Fiber 2.5g
Daily Values: Fiber 10%, Vit C 68%, Vit A 42%, Vit D 5 0%, Calcium 2%, Iron 11%

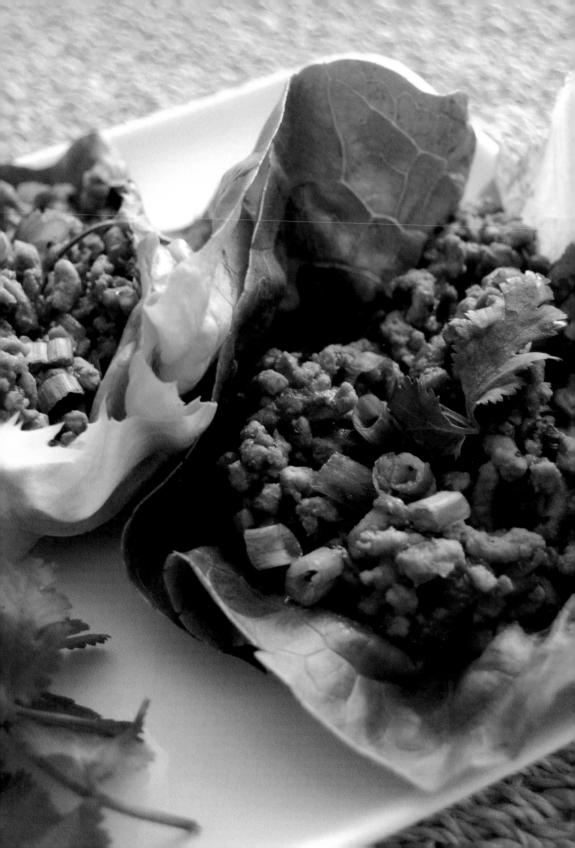

MU SHU PORK–PERUVIAN FUSION LETTUCE CUPS

Servings: 8 ◆ Serving size: 1 lettuce cup

Here Asian meets Latin American in a light and healthy twist on the classic Asian dish—perfect for your belly and waistline.

❶ Heat 1 tablespoon of the oil in a medium-size sauté pan over medium-high heat. Add the pork and cook until browned. Turn off the heat and set aside.

❷ Put the remaining oil in a large sauté pan over medium-high heat. Add the white onion, garlic, and ginger to the pan and cook until soft, for about 5 minutes.

❸ Add the pork, green onion, cilantro, soy sauce, and hoisin sauce to the large sauté pan and sauté until fragrant. Divide the pork filling among the lettuce leaves and top with the sacha inchi seeds before serving.

2 tablespoons canola oil

1 pound extra-lean ground pork

1 small white onion, chopped fine

2 cloves garlic, crushed

1 tablespoon minced fresh ginger

4 green onions, chopped

Handful of fresh cilantro, chopped

2 tablespoons low-sodium soy sauce

2 tablespoons hoisin sauce

8 small lettuce leaves

½ cup crushed, roasted sacha inchi seeds *(or peanuts)*

Per Serving: Kcal 223, Protein 14g, Carb 5g, Fat 16g, Sodium 255mg, Dietary Fiber 1.5g
Daily Values: Fiber 6%, Vit C 6%, Vit A 7%, Vit D 5 3%, Calcium 2%, Iron 5%

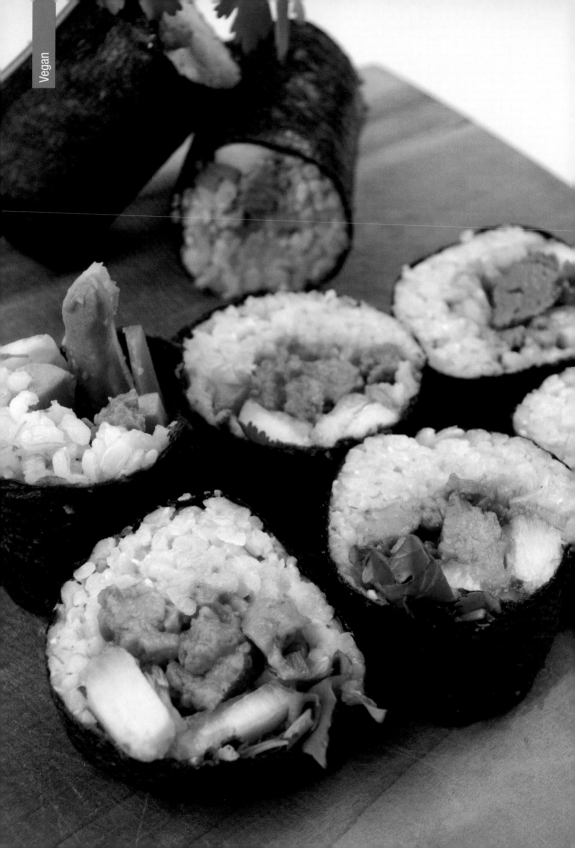

NORI WRAPS À LA PERUVIAN

Servings: 4 ♦ Serving size: One 8-inch-long roll

Sushi, anyone? Our fusion of Japanese and Peruvian flare is fabulous for a lunch on the go.

❶ To make the marinade, put the soy sauce, 2 tablespoons of the vinegar, the garlic, and the ají in a medium bowl. Add the seitan to the bowl; toss with the marinade. Let it marinate at room temperature for 1 hour or in the refrigerator overnight.

❷ While the seitan is marinating, cook the rice. When making sticky brown rice, I like to use a little more water than one might otherwise use. Put the water in a medium saucepan with a lid. Bring to a boil, add the rice, cover, and lower to a simmer for 45 to 50 minutes until most of the water has been absorbed. When the rice is done, but still hot, stir it semi-vigorously for 1 minute to fully incorporate any excess water and make the rice "sticky."

❸ Preheat the oven to 375 degrees F and line a baking sheet with foil.

❹ Measure out 2 cups of the cooked rice and put it in a small bowl with the remaining vinegar. Mix thoroughly. Let the rice cool completely before using.

❺ Drain the marinade from the seitan, reserving it as a dipping sauce for the sushi (keep it in the refrigerator until ready to use). Place the marinated seitan on the baking sheet and bake for 15 minutes, flipping each strip after the first 7 minutes of cooking. Remove from the oven and let it cool completely before using.

¼ cup low-sodium soy sauce

3 tablespoons rice wine vinegar

1 clove garlic, minced

1 tablespoon ají amarillo paste *(or mild chili paste)*

8 ounces *(1 package)* seitan, drained and cut into strips

1 cup brown rice

2⅓ cups water

4 nori seaweed sheets

1 medium carrot, cut into matchsticks

1 medium cucumber, cut into matchsticks

1 avocado, cut into matchsticks

2 tablespoons chopped cilantro

(continued)

⑥ Lay out the nori sheets, placing ½ cup of rice on each sheet. Flatten the rice to form an even layer over each nori sheet, stopping 1½ inches short from the top of the nori sheet.

⑦ Put 1 cup of cold water in a small bowl to assist with the sushi rolling. Set aside.

⑧ Divide the carrot, cucumber, avocado, and cilantro among the four nori sheets to create a level mound in the center of the rice.

⑨ Roll the sushi using a sushi mat (if you do not have a mat, just carefully roll with your fingers) by wrapping the bottom of the nori wrap over the pile of vegetables. Tightly roll up the remainder of the sheet until you reach the 1½-inch portion not covered with rice. Gently dip your fingers in the bowl of cold water and brush them over this portion of the nori, then roll the remaining portion of the sushi to seal. Let it sit for 5 minutes before slicing the roll into 1-inch rounds.

NOTE: Sushi will keep in the refrigerator for two to three days if it is uncut and tightly wrapped in plastic wrap.

Per Serving: Kcal 347.5, Protein 21g, Carb 50g, Fat 8g, Sodium 1385mg, Dietary Fiber 6.5g
Daily Values: Fiber 26%, Vit C 21%, Vit A 62%, Vit D 5 0%, Calcium 6%, Iron 15%

PAPAYA TROPICAL FRUIT SALAD

Servings: 4 ♦ Serving size: ⅝ cup

This fruit salad is refreshing and packed with vitamin C and added protein to keep your skin looking young and renewed.

❶ Put all the ingredients in a medium bowl and toss to combine.

½ cup cubed pineapple

½ cup cubed mango

½ cup cubed papaya

½ cup sliced kiwi

½ cup cubed low-fat queso fresco

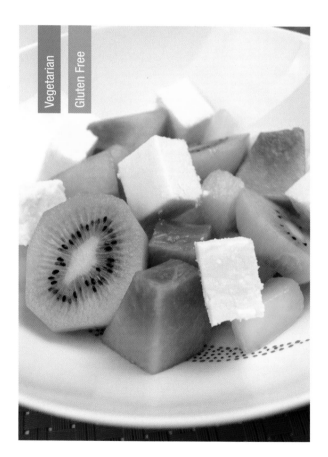

Vegetarian

Gluten Free

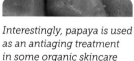

Interestingly, papaya is used as an antiaging treatment in some organic skincare lines. Applied topically, the enzymes help eat away dead skin cells and promote cellular regeneration.

Per Serving: Kcal 88, Protein 4g, Carb 12.5g, Fat 3g, Sodium 42.5mg, Dietary Fiber 1.5g
Daily Values: Fiber 6%, Vit C 77%, Vit A 10%, Vit D 5 0%, Calcium 10%, Iron 2%

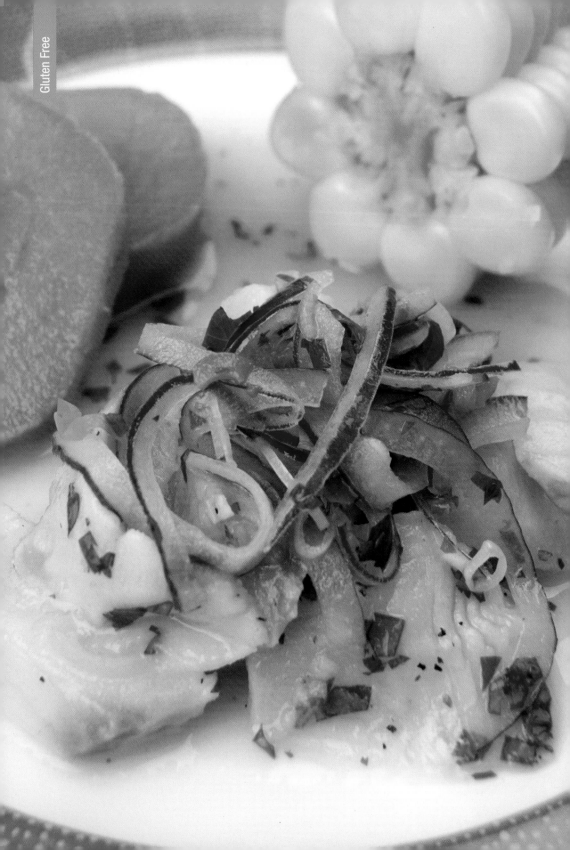

PERUVIAN-STYLE CEVICHE

Servings: 4 ♦ Serving size: ¾ cup

This is one of the most popular dishes in Peru and fabulous for weight loss. Get your protein powered to the max and keep your waistline tight and firm.

❶ Cut the fish into 1-inch pieces and put the pieces in a medium-size bowl with the lime juice, garlic, ají, and cilantro. Toss to combine. Place in the refrigerator, covered, for 15 minutes, then stir the fish mixture and place it back in the refrigerator, covered, for another 15 minutes.

❷ Toss the ceviche with the Salsa Criolla before serving. Eat immediately.

1 pound tilapia or sol

1 cup lime juice

1 clove garlic, crushed

1 tablespoon ají amarillo paste *(or mild chili paste)*

1 tablespoon chopped cilantro

2 cups *(one-half recipe)* Salsa Criolla, prepared without white vinegar *(see recipe on page 253)*

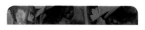

The potassium in cilantro supports cellular health and body fluids that help control heart rate and blood pressure.

Per Serving: Kcal 145, Protein 23.5g, Carb 9.5g, Fat 2g, Sodium 1016mg, Dietary Fiber 0.5g
Daily Values: Fiber 3%, Vit C 38%, Vit A 2%, Vit D 5 0%, Calcium 3%, Iron 4%

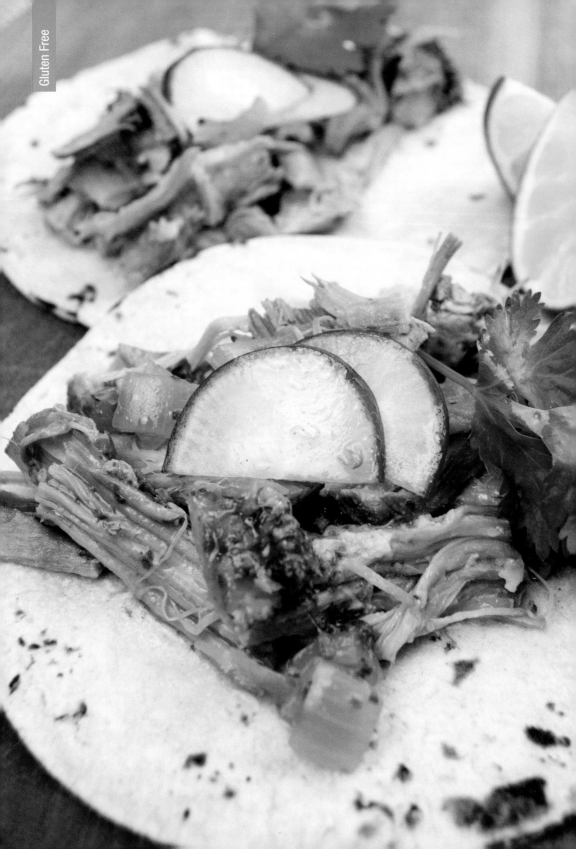

PULLED PORK TACOS

Servings: 12 ◆ Serving size: 1 taco filled with 4 ounces pork

Pork cooked in a crockpot will delicately shred with each touch of a fork. The Peruvian flavors, including cumin, cilantro, and ají, provide all the extra love you need. Prepping this dish only takes three minutes! And cleanup is fast and easy in this one-pot meal.

❶ Put the pork and the chicken stock in the bowl of a slow cooker or crockpot. Cover and put in the refrigerator for 12 hours to marinate.

❷ When the pork is done marinating, combine the garlic, cilantro, cumin, lime juice, and ají in the bowl of a food processer and pulse to form a thick paste.

❸ Add the spice paste and the onion to the bowl with the marinated pork. Season with salt and pepper.

❹ Cook covered on high heat for 8 to 10 hours or until the pork easily shreds when pulled apart with a fork. Serve over corn tortillas.

3 pounds pork tenderloin

8 cups low-sodium chicken stock

3 cloves garlic

1 bunch cilantro

1 tablespoon ground cumin

3 tablespoons lime juice

1 tablespoon ají amarillo paste *(or mild chili paste)*

1 large white onion, minced

Salt and pepper

12 corn tortillas

The cilantro's leaves and stem tips are rich in numerous antioxidant flavonoids that scavenge free radicals and help prevent the onset of heart disease and cancer.

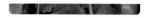

Per Serving: Kcal 252, Protein 30g, Carb 15.5g, Fat 8g, Sodium 330.5mg, Dietary Fiber 2g
Daily Values: Fiber 8%, Vit C 5%, Vit A 2%, Vit D 5 2%, Calcium 6%, Iron 9%

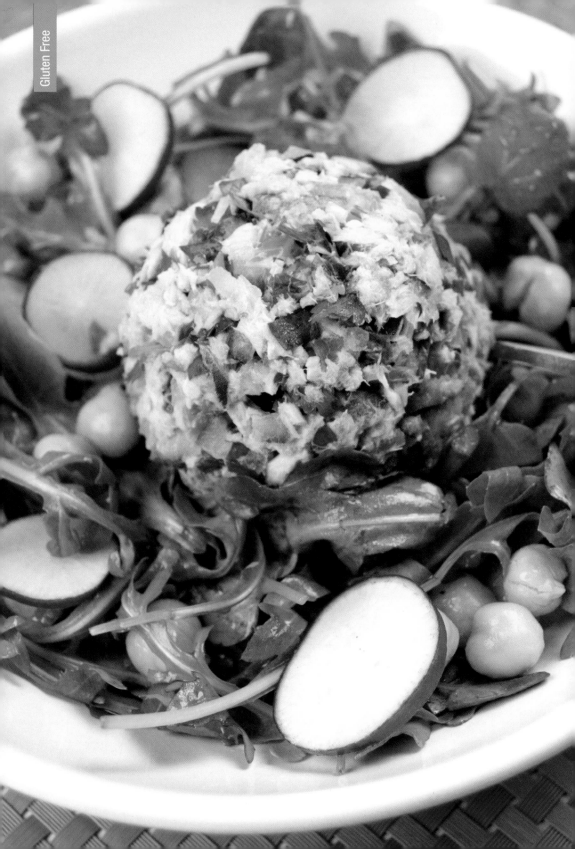

SACHA INCHI SALMON SALAD

Servings: 4 ◆ Serving size: 3 cups

This is a Peruvian twist on the classic tuna salad. We substituted salmon and sacha inchi oil to add extra omega-3s for optimal brain health.

❶ Put the salmon, cilantro, celery, onion, oil, and lime juice in a small bowl and mix to combine. Season with salt and pepper to taste. Set aside.

❷ Put the watercress, arugula, radishes, and garbanzo beans in a separate large bowl. Mix to combine. Top with the salmon salad and serve.

2 cans *(6 ounces each)* salmon, drained

½ cup chopped cilantro

2 medium celery ribs, thinly sliced

½ medium red onion, minced

2 tablespoons sacha inchi oil *(or olive oil)*

¼ cup plus 2 tablespoons lime juice

Salt and pepper

2 cups watercress

6 cups arugula

4 small radishes, thinly sliced

1 can *(15 ounces)* garbanzo beans, drained

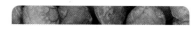

Sacha inchi is a great source of omega-3. There is a strong link between omega-3 fatty acid consumption and healthy brain function. This is because our brains are 60 percent fat, most of which is an omega-3 called DHA. A deficiency of these oils in humans increases the risk for several brain disorders, such as attention deficit disorder, bipolar disorder, dementia, depression, dyslexia, and schizophrenia.

Per Serving: Kcal 143, Protein 33g, Carb 29.5g, Fat 22g,
Sodium 352.5mg, Dietary Fiber 6g
Daily Values: Fiber 24%, Vit C 42%, Vit A 31%, Vit D 5 0%,
Calcium 15%, Iron 19%

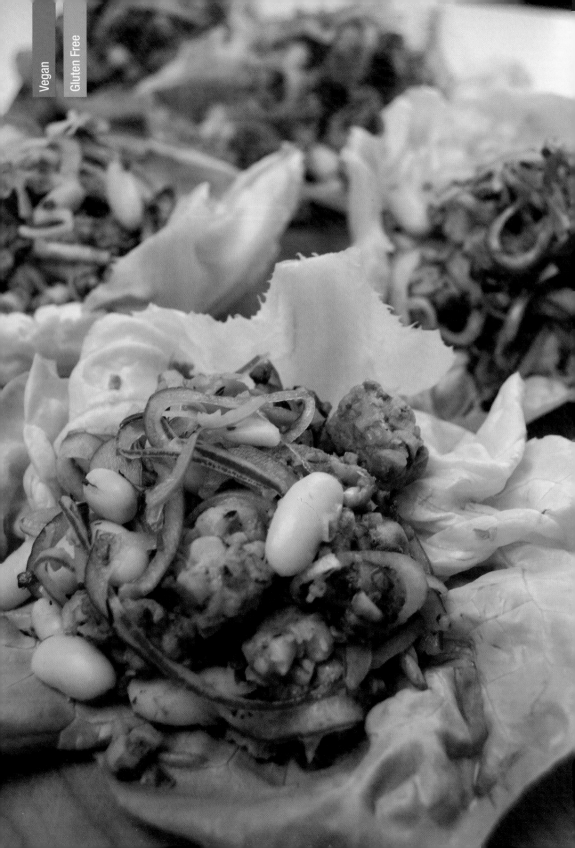

TEMPEH WHITE BEAN CEVICHE LETTUCE CUPS

Servings: 8 ♦ Serving size: 1 lettuce cup

Ceviche is one of the most popular dishes in Lima and worldwide. We thank our friend and chef, Chenoa Bol, for coming up with this lip-smacking and vegan-friendly version using some of our favorite Peruvian flavors. After all, vegans need to enjoy this delicacy, too!

4 cloves garlic, crushed

¼ cup plus 2 tablespoons white vinegar

3 tablespoons Bragg's Liquid Aminos *(or salt)*

2 tablespoons toasted sesame oil

2 tablespoons ají amarillo paste *(or mild chili paste)*

1 teaspoon ground cumin

1 teaspoon dry thyme

16 ounces *(2 packages)* five-grain tempeh, cut into ¾-inch cubes

1 can *(14 ounces)* sodium-free cannellini beans, drained

1 cup Salsa Criolla *(see recipe on page 253)*

1 tablespoon lime juice

Salt and pepper

8 Bibb lettuce leaves

❶ Put the garlic, vinegar, Bragg's, oil, ají paste, cumin, and thyme in a large, shallow bowl. Mix with a fork to create a smooth, homogeneous mixture. Add the tempeh to the marinade and toss to coat. Let it marinate for 30 minutes or overnight in the refrigerator.

❷ Heat a large sauté pan over medium heat. When the pan is hot, add the tempeh with all of the marinade. Cook, stirring often, until the tempeh starts to dry out. When it becomes lightly browned, remove it from the heat and set aside to cool.

❸ In the meantime, put the beans, Salsa Criolla, and lime juice into a large mixing bowl. Add the cooled tempeh to the bowl, along with the salt and pepper to taste. Mix to combine, and then divide the ceviche among the lettuce leaves.

NOTE: Ceviche can be served cold or at room temperature, and it will keep in the refrigerator for three to five days.

Per Serving: Kcal 260.5, Protein 13g, Carb 20g, Fat 7g, Sodium 463.5mg, Dietary Fiber 5.5g
Daily Values: Fiber 22%, Vit C 5%, Vit A 0%, Vit D 5 0%, Calcium 7%, Iron 20%

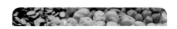

Legumes contain compounds that bolster the immune system to protect against cancers, lower cholesterol levels, and lower blood glucose response.

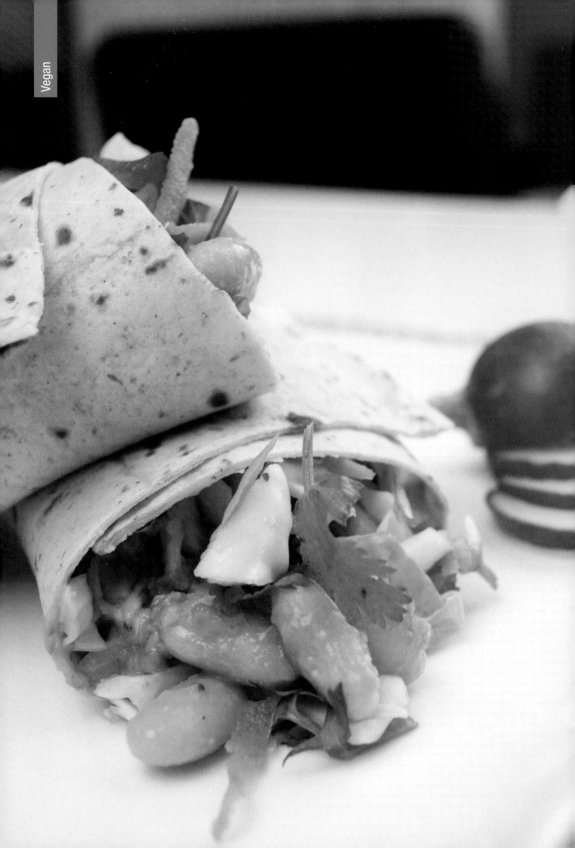

WHITE BEAN AVOCADO WRAP

Servings: 8 ◆ Serving size: ½ wrap

These are fantastic for a light lunch or dinner. You can use the filling on top of a bed of lettuce, too, for a delectable salad. This meal is also vegan.

❶ Put the carrots, cabbage, cilantro, 2 teaspoons of the oil, and 4 teaspoons of the vinegar in a medium bowl. Toss to combine. Season with salt and pepper to taste.

❷ Put the flesh of 1 avocado in a separate medium bowl and mash it with a fork. Add the beans, onion, and remaining oil and vinegar to the avocado mixture. Stir to combine. Season with salt and pepper to taste.

❸ Divide the avocado mixture among the 4 lavash. Top with equal parts of the cabbage slaw and tightly roll each lavash into a wrap. Cut each wrap in half before serving.

4 small carrots, grated

2 cups shredded green cabbage *(about one-quarter head cabbage)*

¼ cup chopped cilantro

4 teaspoons sacha inchi oil *(or olive oil)*

8 teaspoons cider vinegar

Salt and pepper

1 large avocado

2 cups cooked cannellini beans *(see recipe on page 234)*

½ small red onion, minced

4 whole wheat lavash, tortillas, or flatbread

Per Serving: Kcal 158, Protein 8g, Carb 22.5g, Fat 6g, Sodium 297.5mg, Dietary Fiber 9g
Daily Values: Fiber 9%, Vit C 16%, Vit A 78%, Vit D 5 0%, Calcium 7%, Iron 13%

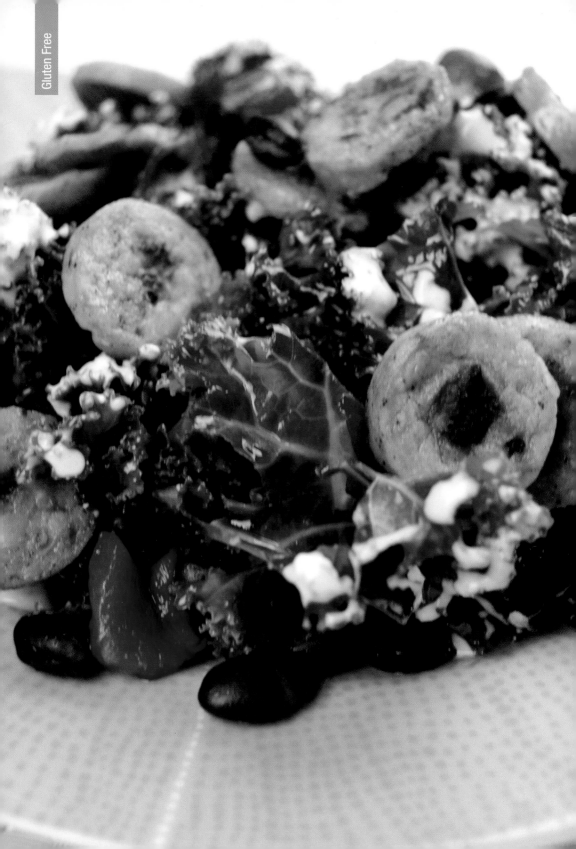

ZESTY KALE & VEGGIE SALAD WITH CHICKEN SAUSAGE

Servings: 4 ◆ Serving size: 3 cups

This powerhouse salad is a complete meal-in-one and super well-balanced with carbohydrates, proteins, and heart-healthy fats. Eating this salad will increase your longevity and vitality. Buen provecho!

❶ Heat the oil in a large sauté pan over medium heat. When the oil is hot, add the sausage and cook until lightly browned, stirring often.

❷ Put the kale, peppers, beans, and sausage in a bowl. Add the dressing and toss to evenly coat the kale leaves. Serve immediately.

2 teaspoons olive oil

4 low-fat chicken sausages, sliced into rounds

8 cups chopped into 1½-inch pieces kale

1 jar *(12 ounces)* roasted red peppers, drained and sliced into 1-inch strips

1 can *(15 ounces)* black beans, drained

½ recipe Zesty Sacha Inchi Cilantro Dressing *(see recipe on page 254)*

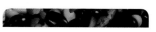

Beans are rich in iron, so they help prevent iron-deficiency anemia, the most common cause of anemia.

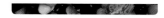

Per Serving: Kcal 397, Protein 29g, Carb 37g, Fat 16g, Sodium 1133mg, Dietary Fiber 8g
Daily Values: Fiber 32%, Vit C 522%, Vit A 469%, Vit D 5 0%, Calcium 26%, Iron 28%

ZESTY VEGAN CHICKPEA SALAD

Servings: 4 ♦ Serving size: 1 cup

2 cans *(15 ounces each)* chickpeas, drained

2 large celery ribs, minced

¼ cup chopped fresh dill

¼ cup vegan mayo

2 tablespoons brown mustard

Salt and pepper

Jamie Farnsworth, vegan and founder of the blog Girl Eats Greens (girleatsgreens.com), gave us this amazing, mouthwatering recipe. Her blog is off the hook and full of delicious vegan recipes for all.

❶ Put all the ingredients in a large bowl. Using a potato masher, mash the chickpeas until they break down but still have some texture (the occasional whole chickpea isn't a bad thing).

NOTE: This salad is good served with avocado slices and lettuce in whole wheat pita bread. Enjoy and be prepared to be full!

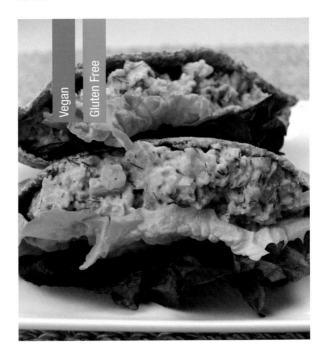

Per Serving: Kcal 302.5, Protein 11g, Carb 52g, Fat 6g, Sodium 1138.5mg, Dietary Fiber 10g
Daily Values: Fiber 40%, Vit C 15%, Vit A 4%, Vit D 5 0%, Calcium 9%, Iron 18%

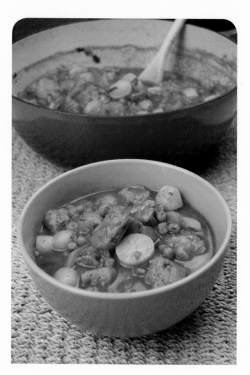

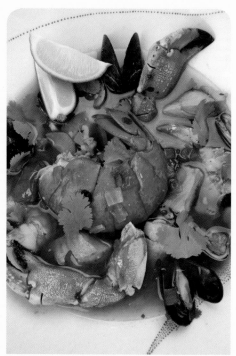

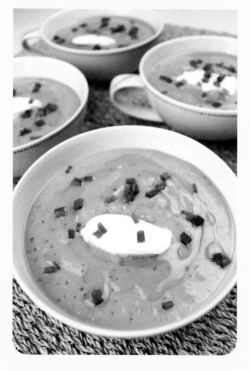

Soups, Stews & Curries

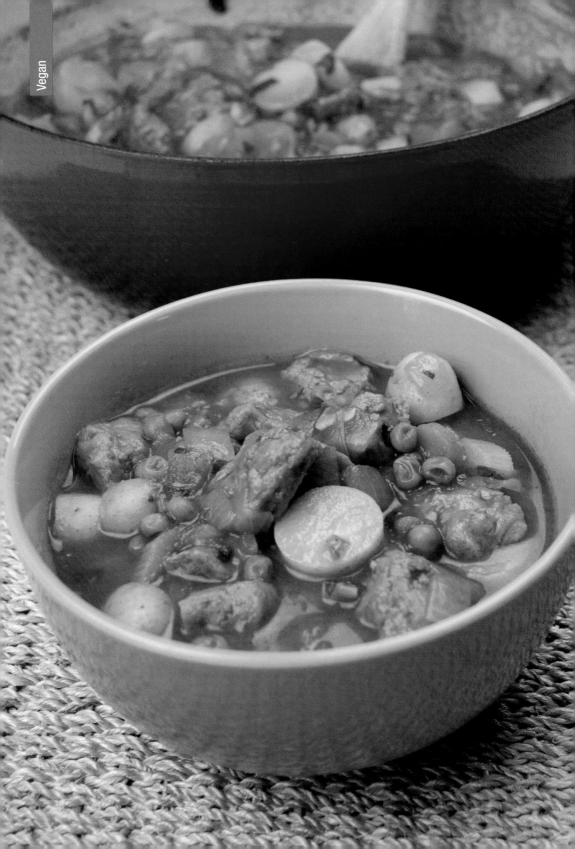

ESTOFADO DE SEITAN

Servings: 5 ◆ Serving size: 2 cups

"Estofado" is a Peruvian word for "stews" and is a common family dish. Normally, estofado is made with "pollo" (chicken). However, in this delectable vegan version, we kept all of the taste and the protein in a new fusion of "sabor" (flavor).

❶ Heat the oil in a Dutch oven or large soup pot over low heat. When the oil is hot, add the onion, garlic, carrots, and seitan. Sauté for 5 minutes or until the onions begin to wilt.

❷ Add the ají, cumin, and the tomato paste to the pot. Stir to combine. When fragrant, add the potatoes and vegetable broth.

❸ Raise the heat to medium-high and cover the pot with a lid. When the stew comes to a boil, lower and simmer, covered, for 30 minutes. Stir occasionally.

❹ Add the green peas and the parsley to the pot. Season with salt and pepper. Continue cooking, uncovered, for 15 minutes or to desired consistency.

2 tablespoons canola oil of choice

1 medium yellow onion, coarsely chopped

2 cloves garlic, minced

2 medium carrots, sliced into ¼-inch rounds

16 ounces *(1 package)* seitan, cubed

1 tablespoon ají amarillo paste *(or mild chili paste)*

1 teaspoon cumin powder

¼ cup tomato paste

1 pound yellow potatoes, cut into 1-inch cubes

4 cups vegetable broth

1 cup frozen green peas

½ cup chopped fresh parsley

Salt and pepper

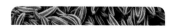

Cumin seeds are an excellent source of iron, a very good source of manganese, and a good source of calcium, magnesium, phosphorus, and vitamin B.

Per Serving: Kcal 321, Protein 25.5g, Carb 38.5g, Fat 8g, Sodium 1020mg, Dietary Fiber 5g
Daily Values: Fiber 21%, Vit C 58%, Vit A 97%, Vit D 5 0%, Calcium 8%, Iron 28%

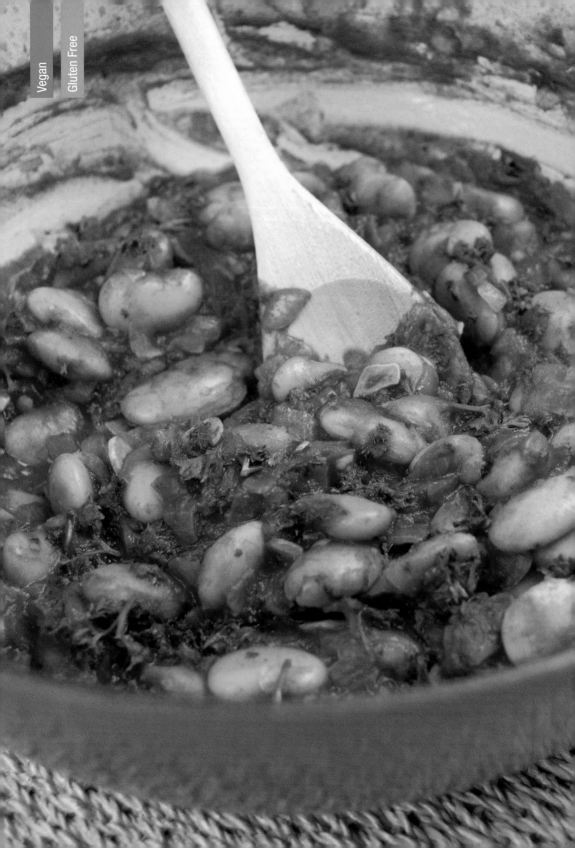

LIMA BEAN STEW

Servings: 5 ◆ Serving size: 1 cup

Get ready to experience a traditional lima bean stew infused with Peruvian flavors. This is great for lunch or leftovers any day of the week.

❶ Heat the oil in a large saucepan over medium heat. When the oil is hot, add the onion and garlic. Sauté until soft and fragrant. Stir in the ají and paprika and cook for another minute.

❷ Add the water, tomato sauce, and lima beans to the pan and cook, uncovered, over low heat, making sure to stir the pot every few minutes. Season with salt and pepper to taste. Toss with the fresh parsley before serving.

1 tablespoon olive oil

1 medium yellow onion, diced

4 cloves garlic, sliced

2 tablespoons ají panca paste *(or mild chili paste)*

½ teaspoon smoked paprika

1 cup water

1 cup tomato sauce

2 jars *(12 ounces each)* lima beans *(or 3 cups frozen)*

Salt and pepper

½ cup chopped parsley

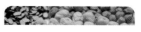

Fiber from legumes improves blood sugar levels and insulin sensitivity in nondiabetic and diabetic individuals. Fiber can also significantly enhance weight loss efforts.

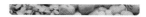

Per Serving: Kcal 174, Protein 8.5g, Carb 30.5g, Fat 3g, Sodium 995mg, Dietary Fiber 6.5g
Daily Values: Fiber 25%, Vit C 28%, Vit A 16%, Vit D 5 0%, Calcium 5%, Iron 14%

Vegan

Gluten Free

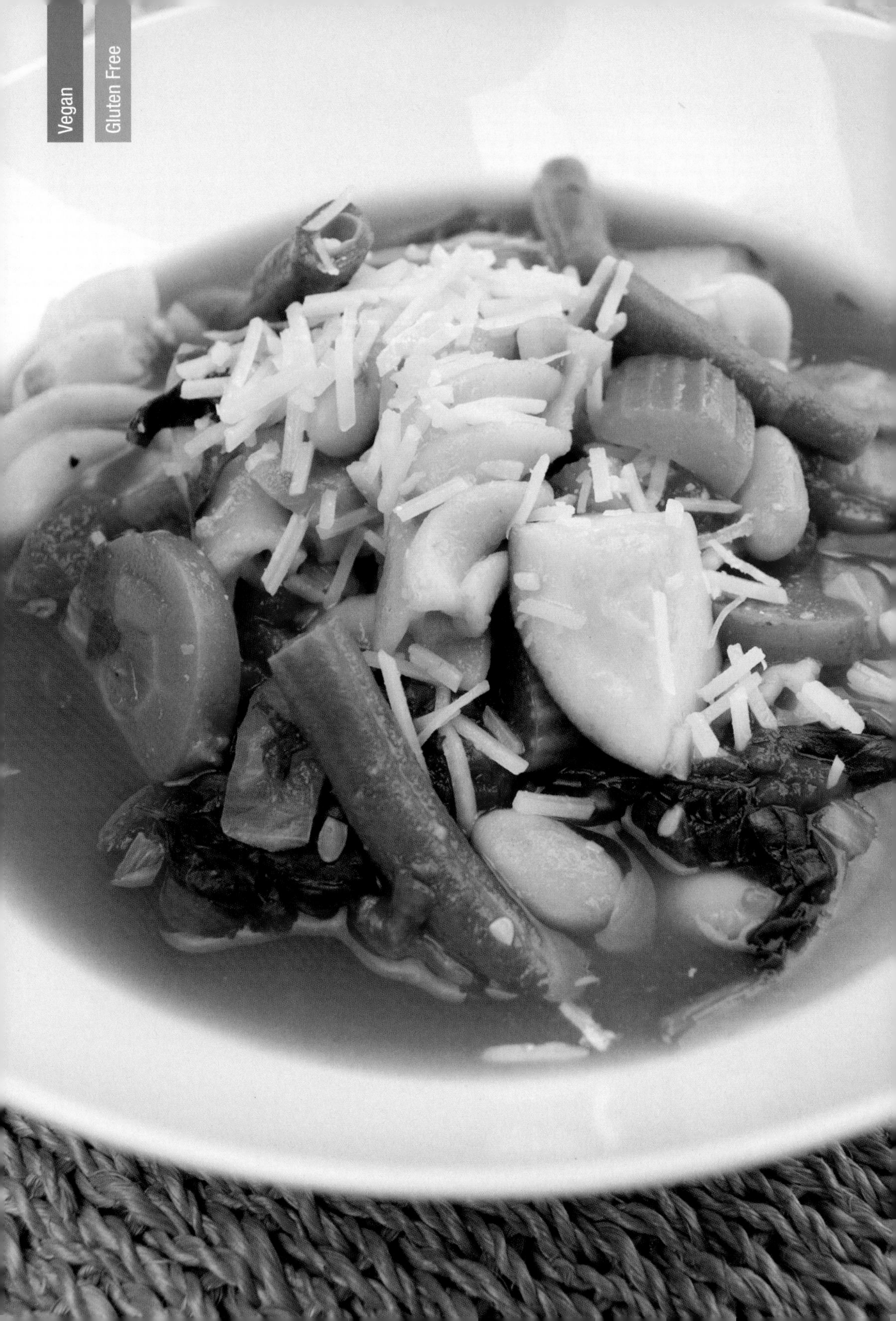

MINESTRONE WITH QUINOA NOODLES

Servings: 8 ◆ Serving size: 1½ cups

This is a Peruvian-infused twist on the classic Italian soup. You get extra protein from the quinoa noodles and cannellini beans. This meal is gluten-free, too.

❶ Heat the oil in a Dutch oven or large stockpot over medium heat. When the oil is hot, add the garlic and onion and cook until fragrant, of about 2 minutes. Add the celery and carrots and cook for another 3 to 5 minutes.

❷ Add the broth, beans, tomatoes, zucchini, spinach, green beans, bay leaves, and parsley to the pot. Season with salt and pepper to taste. Bring the contents of the pot to a boil, then reduce the heat to a simmer. Cook, covered, for 30 minutes.

❸ Add the pasta and cook for another 10 minutes or until the pasta is al dente. Serve with 1 tablespoon Parmesan cheese sprinkled on top.

*The Parmesan cheese is not included in the nutrient analysis.

2 teaspoons olive oil

2 cloves garlic, crushed

1 large white onion, chopped

2 large celery ribs, sliced

2 large carrots, sliced

3 cups reduced-sodium vegetable broth

1 can *(15 ounces)* cannellini beans

1 can *(28 ounces)* diced tomatoes

1 large zucchini, sliced

1 bunch spinach

1 cup fresh green beans, cut into 1-inch pieces

2 bay leaves

¼ cup chopped parsley

Salt and pepper

2 cups quinoa pasta

½ cup shredded Parmesan cheese *(optional)**

Phytosterols from quinoa have anti-inflammatory effects, making quinoa a potentially great food for people experiencing diseases such as arthritis, metabolic syndrome, or the many gastrointestinal inflammatory diseases.

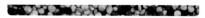

Per Serving: Kcal 236, Protein 5.5g, Carb 33g, Fat 1.5g, Sodium 719.5mg, Dietary Fiber 7.5g
Daily Values: Fiber 30%, Vit C 43%, Vit A 75%, Vit D 5 0%, Calcium 11%, Iron 15%

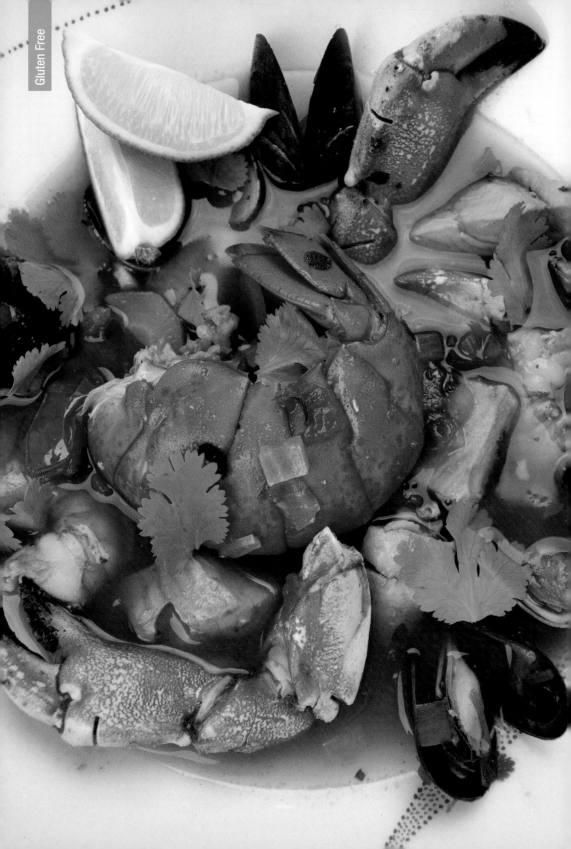

PERUVIAN SEAFOOD SOUP

Servings: 4 ◆ Serving size: 3 cups

Experience the traditional Peruvian seafood soup similar to the classic Italian seafood soup, cioppino. You will immediately be transported on a Peruvian epicurean adventure.

❶ Heat the oil in a Dutch oven over medium heat. When the oil is hot, add the onion and garlic, and cook until translucent, for about 3 minutes.

❷ Add the tomato, carrots, paprika, ají panca, ají amarillo, cumin, oregano, and wine to the onion mixture. Cook for a few minutes until fragrant. Season with salt and pepper to taste.

❸ Add the crab, shrimp, mussels, clams, cod, and cilantro to the pot, along with 6 cups of the fish broth. Bring the soup to a boil, then turn off the heat. Cover the pot and allow the soup to steep for 10 minutes before serving with lime wedges.

1 tablespoon canola oil

1 medium yellow onion, diced

4 cloves garlic, crushed

1 medium tomato, chopped

4 medium carrots, sliced into rounds

1 tablespoon ground paprika

1 tablespoon ají panca paste *(or mild chili paste)*

3 tablespoons ají amarillo paste *(or mild chili paste)*

1 teaspoon ground cumin

1 tablespoon dried oregano

¾ cup white wine

Salt and pepper

4 crab claws, cleaned

4 shrimp, cleaned

8 mussels, cleaned

8 clams, cleaned

8 ounces cod or sea bass, cut into 1-inch pieces

¼ cup chopped cilantro

6 cups fish stock

1 to 2 limes, cut into wedges for garnish

Per Serving: Kcal 271, Protein 26.5g, Carb 15g, Fat 8g, Sodium 968mg, Dietary Fiber 3.5g
Daily Values: Fiber 14%, Vit C 30%, Vit A 230%, Vit D 5 44%, Calcium 9%, Iron 32%

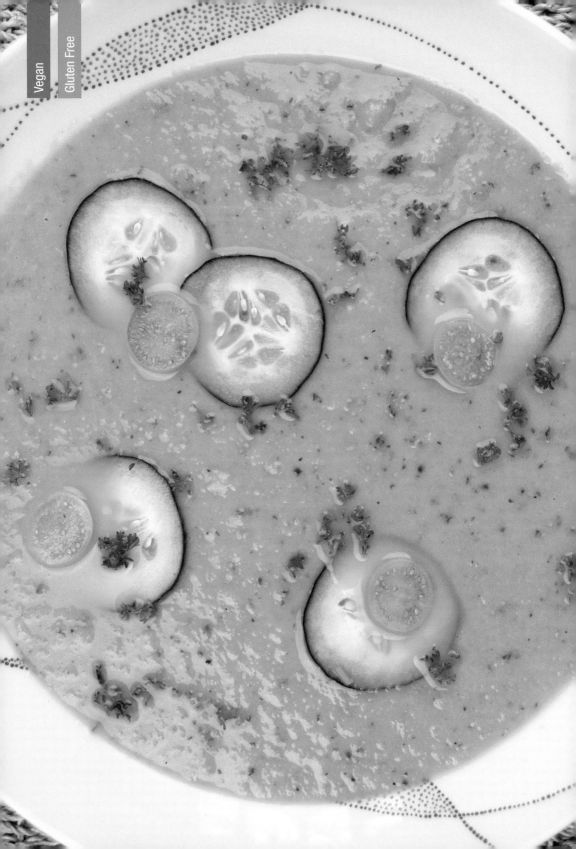

PICHUBERRY GAZPACHO

Servings: 4 ♦ Serving size: 2 cups

Gazpacho is a traditional Andalusian chilled tomato soup from Spain. We infused this gazpacho with Peruvian power foods, such as pichuberries, for an extra vitamin C punch.

❶ Put the onion, bell pepper, cucumber, carrot, celery, tomatoes, garlic, parsley, and 1 cup of the pichuberries in a large bowl. Toss to combine.

❷ In a separate bowl, combine the vegetable stock, lime juice, vinegar, and oil.

❸ Put half of the vegetable mixture and half of the liquids in a blender and puree. Repeat with the remaining vegetables and liquids. Add salt and pepper to taste.

❹ Refrigerate for 1 hour before serving to let the flavors marinate. Adjust the salt and pepper if necessary.

❺ Slice the remaining cup of pichuberries and add to the gazpacho just before serving.

½ medium red onion, chopped

1 medium green bell pepper, chopped

1 medium cucumber, chopped

1 medium carrot, chopped

2 medium celery ribs, chopped

2 large Roma tomatoes, chopped

1 clove garlic, crushed

½ cup chopped parsley

2 cups pichuberries

3 cups vegetable stock

Juice of 1 lime *(about 1½ to 2 tablespoons)*

2 tablespoons white wine vinegar

2 tablespoons olive oil

Salt and pepper

Per Serving: Kcal 160.5, Protein 3g, Carb 22g, Fat 7g, Sodium 174.5mg, Dietary Fiber 4g
Daily Values: Fiber 16%, Vit C 87%, Vit A 99%, Vit D 5 26%, Calcium 7%, Iron 7%

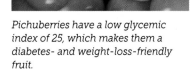

Pichuberries have a low glycemic index of 25, which makes them a diabetes- and weight-loss-friendly fruit.

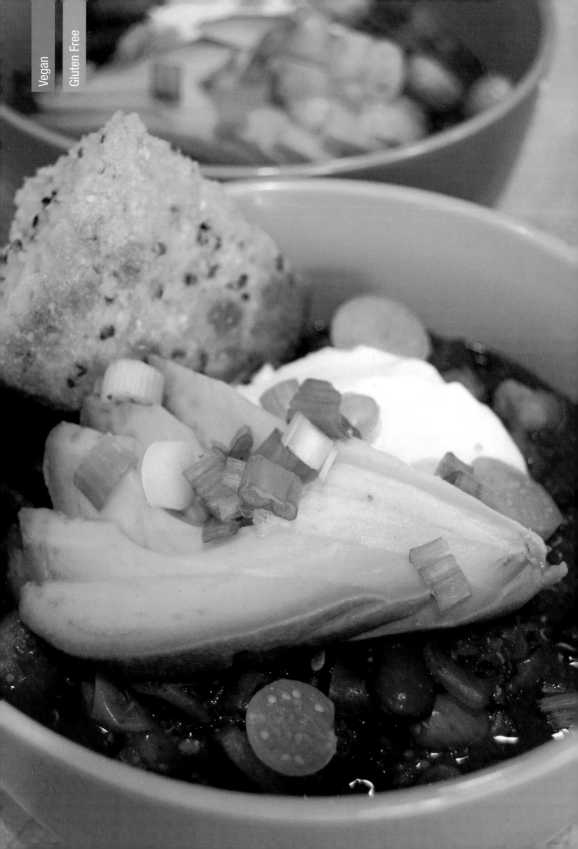

PICHUBERRY QUINOA CHILI

Servings: 8 ♦ Serving size: 1½ cups

We fused this American classic with a Peruvian flare by adding the super of the superfruits, pichuberry.

❶ Heat the oil in a large stockpot over medium heat. Add the onion and cook until soft, for about 5 minutes. Add the jalapeño, carrot, celery, bell pepper, zucchini, and garlic to the pot. Cook, stirring often, until the vegetables start to soften, for about 10 minutes.

❷ Stir in the pichuberries and cook for another 3 to 5 minutes, until they start releasing some of their juices.

❸ Add the quinoa, water, beans (along with their liquids), canned tomatoes with juice, cumin, chili powder, oregano, smoked paprika, salt, and pepper to taste. Stir to combine.

❹ Cover the pot and let the chili simmer on low heat for 25 to 30 minutes until fragrant. Serve warm, with your choice of toppings.

NOTE: Serve the chili with your choice of optional toppings (accompaniments are not included in the nutrient analysis).

Per Serving: Kcal 315, Protein 12g, Carb 55.5g, Fat 5.5g,
Sodium 545mg, Dietary Fiber 51g
Daily Values: Fiber 51%, Vit C 50%, Vit A 86%, Vit D 5 13%,
Calcium 9%, Iron 16%

2 tablespoons canola oil

1 medium yellow onion, diced in ½-inch pieces

1 small jalapeño, seeded and minced

2 large carrots, diced in ½-inch pieces

2 medium ribs celery, diced in ½-inch pieces

1 medium green bell pepper, diced in ½-inch pieces

1 large zucchini, diced in ½-inch pieces

4 cloves garlic, minced

2 cups pichuberries, halved

½ cup quinoa

1 cup water

1 can *(15 ounces)* black beans with liquid

1 can *(15 ounces)* kidney beans with liquid

1 can *(15 ounces)* canary beans *(or pinto beans)* with liquid

1 can *(15 ounces)* diced tomatoes

1 tablespoon ground cumin

2 tablespoons chili powder

2 teaspoons dry oregano

1 teaspoon ground smoked paprika

Salt and pepper

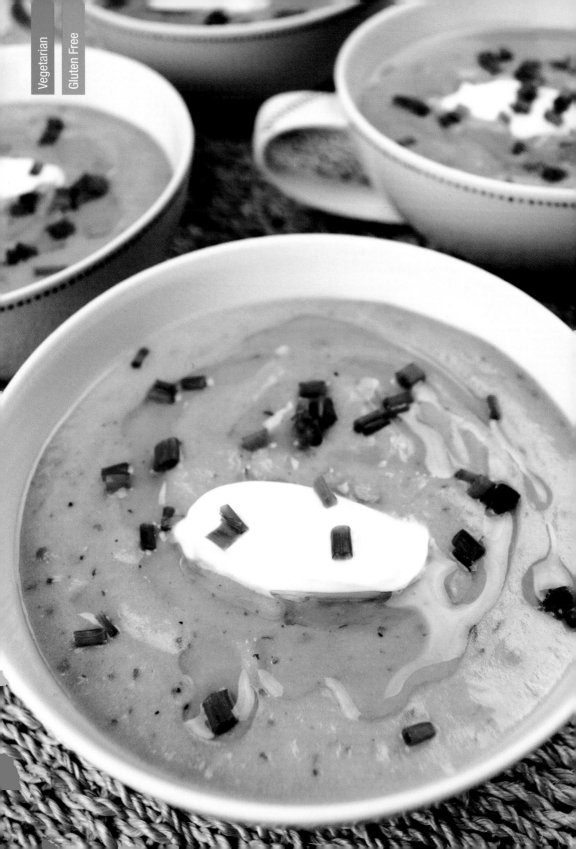

PURPLE POTATO LEEK SOUP

Servings: 8 ◆ Serving size: 1 cup

Prepare this soup on the weekend so you have lunch ready to go throughout the week.

❶ Heat the oil in a large Dutch oven over medium heat. When the oil is hot, add the leeks and sauté for 5 minutes or until wilted and slightly caramelized.

❷ Add the potatoes, milk, bay leaves, thyme, and paprika. Cover and let simmer on very low heat until the potatoes are soft, for 15 to 20 minutes, stirring every 5 minutes to prevent burning. Let the soup cool for 10 minutes before moving on to the next step.

❸ Remove the bay leaves and puree the soup using a handheld blender. The soup can also be transferred to a countertop blender and pureed in batches.

❹ Add the Parmesan cheese and salt and pepper to taste. Garnish with a dollop of nonfat Greek yogurt and chives just before serving.

The yogurt and chives are not included in the nutrient analysis.

2 tablespoons olive oil

4 large leeks, sliced, then washed

1½ pounds purple potatoes, sliced into ½-inch rounds

6 cups low-fat milk

2 bay leaves

1 teaspoon dried thyme

½ teaspoon smoked paprika

¾ cup grated Parmesan cheese

Salt and pepper

Minced chives and nonfat Greek yogurt for garnish*

Per Serving: Kcal 237.5, Protein 12g, Carb 31g, Fat 7.5g, Sodium 500mg, Dietary Fiber 2g
Daily Values: Fiber 8%, Vit C 9%, Vit A 24%, Vit D 5 24%, Calcium 33%, Iron 8%

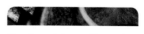

Purple potatoes offer an array of essential nutrients, including complex carbohydrates, folic acid, potassium, and vitamin C.

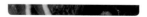

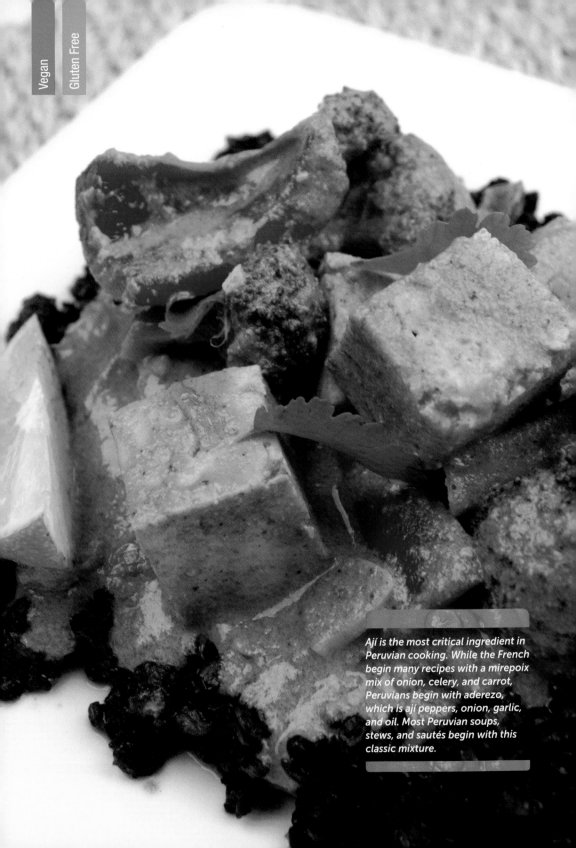

Ají is the most critical ingredient in Peruvian cooking. While the French begin many recipes with a mirepoix mix of onion, celery, and carrot, Peruvians begin with aderezo, which is ají peppers, onion, garlic, and oil. Most Peruvian soups, stews, and sautés begin with this classic mixture.

TOFU VEGETABLE AJÍ PANCA CURRY

Servings: 8 ◆ Serving size: 1 cup

This flavor-packed curry comes to us from our colleague, chef, and curry enthusiast, Chenoa Bol. Although coconut milk is not an ingredient commonly used in Peruvian cuisine, it pairs beautifully with the roasted spiciness of ají panca chili paste.

① Heat 2 teaspoons of the oil in a large sauté pan over medium heat. When the oil is hot, add the tofu and 2 teaspoons of the curry powder and cook until nicely browned, for about 5 minutes. Season with salt and pepper to taste. Set aside.

② Combine the water, coconut milk, tahini, ají, and agave in a medium-size bowl and set aside.

③ Heat the remaining oil in a Dutch oven over medium heat. When the oil is hot, add the onion, bell pepper, carrots, and broccoli and cook until fragrant, for about 5 minutes. Add the ginger and garlic and sauté for another 2 to 3 minutes. Season with the remaining curry powder and salt and pepper to taste.

④ Add the tofu and coconut milk slurry to the pot and simmer over low heat for 5 to 7 minutes until slightly thickened and fragrant.

⑤ Serve the curry over rice with cilantro sprinkled on top.

NOTE: The curry will keep in the refrigerator for three to five days.

Per Serving: Kcal 139, Protein 5.5g, Carb 11g, Fat 9g, Sodium 394.5mg, Dietary Fiber 2.5g
Daily Values: Fiber 10%, Vit C 50%, Vit A 63%, Vit D 5 0%, Calcium 13%, Iron 9%

4 teaspoons canola oil

1 block *(14 ounces)* **extra-firm tofu, cut into 1-inch pieces**

4 teaspoons curry powder

Salt and pepper

1 cup water

1 can *(13.5 ounces)* light coconut milk

2 tablespoons tahini

¼ cup plus 2 tablespoons ají panca paste *(or mild chili paste)*

1 teaspoon agave syrup

1 large red onion, cut into 1-inch pieces

1 large red bell pepper, cut into 1-inch pieces

2 medium carrots, cut into ½-inch-thick slices

½ head broccoli, cut into 1-inch pieces

2 tablespoons minced fresh ginger

6 cloves garlic, sliced

Handful of fresh cilantro, chopped

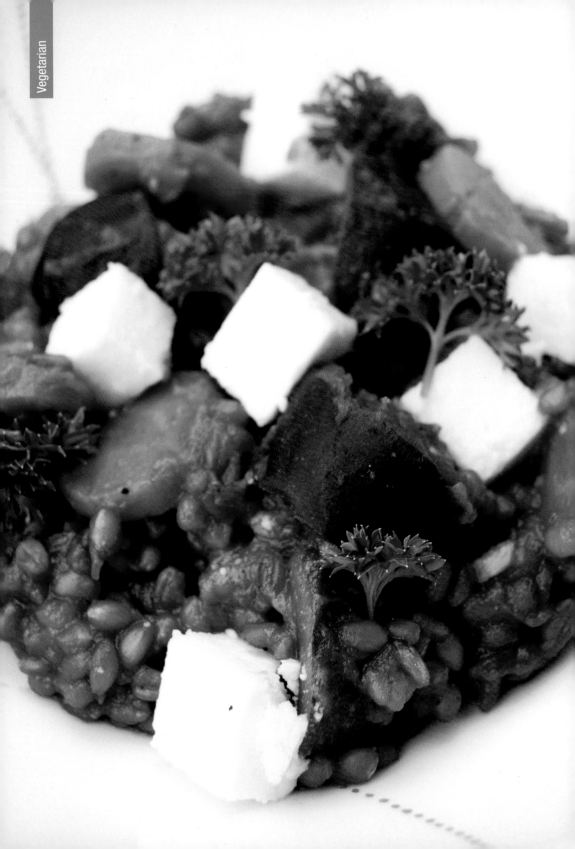

TRIGO GUISADO

"Trigo" is the word for wheat berries, which are very popular in the Andes of Peru and nationwide. Guisado is like a stew. This stew will warm your heart and soul and satisfy every bone in your body.

❶ Put the wheat berries in a medium bowl with enough cold water to cover by 2 inches. Let them soak for 8 hours or overnight, then drain.

❷ Heat the oil in a medium-size saucepan over medium heat. When the oil is hot, add the onion and garlic and cook until nicely browned, for about 5 minutes.

❸ Add the tomato paste, ají, potatoes, broth, and wheat berries. Cover and simmer over low heat for 40 to 60 minutes, stirring occasionally, until the wheat is tender.

❹ Remove from the heat and stir in the queso fresco. Season with salt and pepper to taste.

1½ cups wheat berries

2 teaspoons olive oil

1 large yellow onion, diced

3 cloves garlic, minced

¼ cup tomato paste

1 tablespoon ají panca paste *(or mild chili paste)*

12 ounces purple potatoes, cut into 1-inch cubes

8 cups vegetable broth

1 package *(10 ounces)* part skim milk queso fresco, cut into ½-inch cubes

Salt and pepper

Per Serving: Kcal 329, Protein 14g, Carb 55g, Fat 6g, Sodium 774.5mg, Dietary Fiber 9g
Daily Values: Fiber 36%, Vit C 7%, Vit A 8%, Vit D 5 0%, Calcium 19%, Iron 15%

WHOLESOME ROASTED EGGPLANT STEW

Servings: 4 ♦ Serving size: 2 cups

2 tablespoons olive oil

1 medium red onion, diced

6 cloves garlic, minced

2 small Italian eggplants, cut into 1-inch cubes

3 large carrots, sliced

2 large celery ribs, sliced

1 teaspoon ground cumin

1 can *(6 ounces)* tomato paste

2 cups low-sodium beef broth

1 cup red cooking wine

1 pound lean beef, cubed

Salt and pepper

Handful of chopped parsley for garnish

Roasted eggplant beef stew truly comes from the heart and is one of my mother's secret recipes. Growing up, she would make it for us often, and, every time we ate it, our souls would be happy, wholesome, and warm. No matter what I do, the recipe never tastes the same as when my mom cooks it, but it is definitely delicious and will rock your world with homemade comfort food. Thank you, Mom, for allowing me to share this secret with everyone. We all love your cooking!

❶ Heat the oil in a large Dutch oven over medium heat. When the oil is hot, add the onion and garlic. Sauté until soft and fragrant, for about 5 minutes. Stir in the eggplant, carrots, celery, and cumin and cook for another 5 minutes.

❷ Add the tomato paste, broth, wine, and beef to the pot. Reduce the heat to a simmer and let cook, covered, for 45 minutes. Stir the stew every 10 minutes. Add salt and pepper to taste.

❸ Garnish with the parsley before serving.

Per Serving: Kcal 455, Protein 32g, Carb 36.5g, Fat 17g, Sodium 1086.5mg, Dietary Fiber 13.5g
Daily Values: Fiber 54%, Vit C 45%, Vit A 176%, Vit D 5 2%, Calcium 11%, Iron 30%

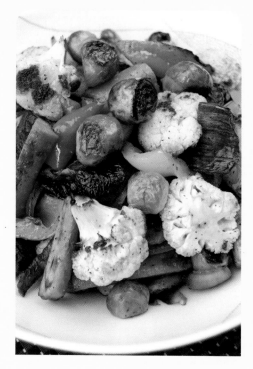

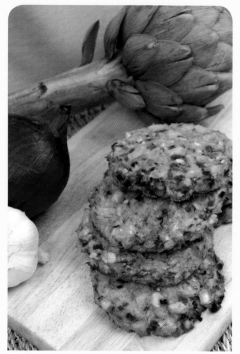

Snacks & Sides

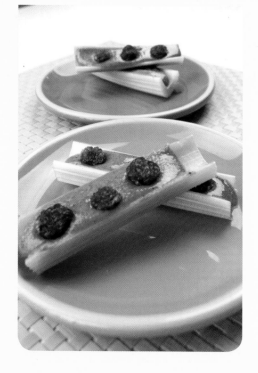

ANTS ON A LOG, PERUVIAN STYLE

Servings: 6 ♦ Serving size: One-third celery rib

2 large celery ribs

¼ cup sacha inchi butter
(or almond butter)

24 dried pichuberries
(or raisins)

A Peruvian-inspired twist on the classic American after-school snack. Fabulous for both adults and kids, this snack is for fueling your brain for the rest of the afternoon.

❶ Cut each celery rib into three pieces of equal size. Fill each piece of celery with 2 teaspoons of sacha inchi butter. Distribute the dried pichuberries among the celery sticks (4 berries per log) so that they sit on top of the sacha inchi butter.

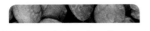

Sacha inchi is a singular power food, providing the highest levels of omega-3 fatty acids in any plant on the planet! It was so cherished in Incan civilization that representations of the plant and its fruits have been found in Incan tombs.

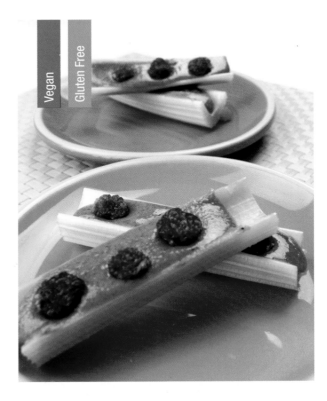

Per Serving: Kcal 103, Protein 4.5g, Carb 5g, Fat 7g, Sodium 43mg, Dietary Fiber 2g
Daily Values: Fiber 8%, Vit C 1%, Vit A 9%, Vit D 5 0%, Calcium 1%, Iron 1%

BAKED SWEET POTATO FRIES WITH COCONUT OIL

Servings: 4 ♦ Serving size: ½ sweet potato

Fries go with almost anything! Take pleasure in this low-fat baked version of fries made with sweet potatoes for extra health and wellness.

2 large sweet potatoes

Coconut oil spray

Salt and pepper

❶ Preheat the oven to 400 degrees F.

❷ Wash the sweet potatoes and pat dry. Slice them lengthwise into ½-inch-thick sticks.

❸ Place the sweet potato sticks on a large baking sheet and spray them with coconut oil to coat. Season with salt and pepper to taste.

❹ Bake for 20 to 30 minutes, flipping once halfway through the baking process, until the fries are golden in color. Serve warm.

NOTE: Fries are best eaten on the day they are made.

Vegan

Gluten Free

Sweet potatoes are potent free radical scavengers that prevent DNA damage at the cellular level, helping to prevent disease and to slow aging.

Per Serving: Kcal 61, Protein 1g, Carb 13g, Fat 0.5g, Sodium 36mg, Dietary Fiber 2g
Daily Values: Fiber 8%, Vit C 3%, Vit A 0%, Vit D 5 0%, Calcium 2%, Iron 2%

CAPRESE PICHUBERRY SKEWERS

Servings: 12 ♦ Serving size: 1 skewer

12 pichuberries

12 baby low-fat mozzarella balls

12 small basil leaves

12 toothpicks or small wooden skewers

These are perfect for a fancy party or a simple snack. When I think of hors d'oeuvres, the first thing that comes to mind is the pichuberry. With its sweet yet tart flavor in a bite-size package, it complements both sweet and savory palates equally. Wow everyone's taste buds with this exotic delicacy.

❶ Make the skewers by putting a pichuberry, a mozzarella ball, and a basil leaf on a toothpick or small wooden skewer.

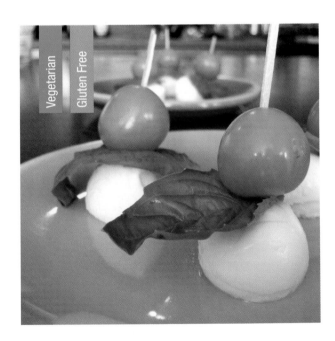

The whole pichuberry contains oil that is rich in fifteen fatty acids, including linoleic acid, an essential oil that cannot be produced by humans.

Per Serving: Kcal 64, Protein 2.5g, Carb 8g, Fat 2.5g, Sodium 33.5mg, Dietary Fiber 0.5g
Daily Values: Fiber 2%, Vit C 38%, Vit A 22%, Vit D 5 22%, Calcium 4%, Iron 0%

INCA POWER BARS

Servings: 12 ♦ Serving size: 1 bar

These wholesome, homemade energy bars are superfilling and power-packed with antioxidants and protein to keep you energized and fueled.

❶ Put all the ingredients in a small bowl and toss to combine. Working in batches, grind the mixture in a food processor to form a coarse, homogeneous paste.

❷ Press the paste into a parchment-lined baking dish. Put a second piece of parchment paper over the top of the paste and press down with your hands to ensure a smooth, uniform surface.

❸ Put the paste in the refrigerator for 1 hour. Once it has hardened, cut it into twelve bars using a chef's knife.

NOTE: The bars can be stored in the refrigerator for up to a week.

½ cup dried pichuberries

½ cup cacao nibs

½ cup sacha inchi seeds *(or peanuts)*

½ cup unsweetened coconut

½ cup halved and pitted dates

¼ cup yacon syrup *(or agave syrup)*

Vegan | Gluten Free

Per Serving: Kcal 108, Protein 3g, Carb 15.5g, Fat 5.5g, Sodium 9.5mg, Dietary Fiber 3.5g
Daily Values: Fiber 14%, Vit C 1%, Vit A 8%, Vit D 5 0%, Calcium 1%, Iron 3%

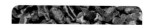

Cacao flavonols are scientifically proven to help support healthy circulation by helping your arteries stay supple. Cacao has also been shown to build resistance to oxidative stress, which can cause inflammation and atherosclerosis. For this reason, cacao is a phenomenal antiaging agent.

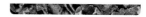

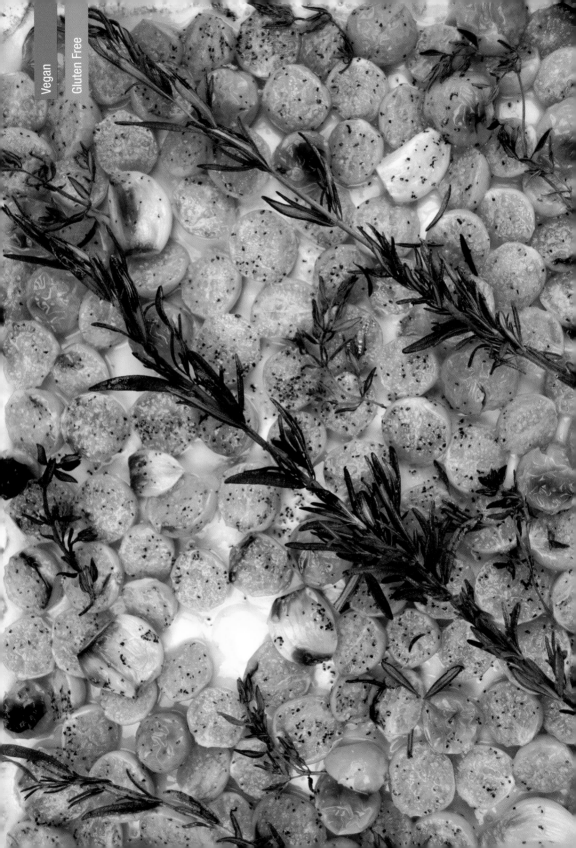

OVEN-ROASTED PICHUBERRIES

Servings: 4 ♦ Serving size: ¼ cup

This recipe was inspired by oven-roasted tomatoes. Use these as a side dish or a condiment, or put them on top of rice, quinoa, tofu, or eggs. They are also perfect for enhancing foods that are slightly bland by bringing a burst of tart flavor.

4 cups pichuberries, halved

6 cloves garlic

1 tablespoon olive oil

10 sprigs fresh thyme

3 sprigs fresh rosemary

Salt and pepper

❶ Preheat the oven to 400 degrees F.

❷ Place the pichuberries, cut side up, in a large baking dish. Evenly distribute the whole garlic cloves among the pichuberries. Drizzle with the olive oil. Distribute the herb sprigs over the surface of the pichuberries along with salt and pepper to taste.

❸ Bake for 10 to 15 minutes or until the pichuberries start to shrivel but still hold their shape. Let them cool slightly before using.

NOTE: The pichuberries will keep in the refrigerator for up to three days.

Phytochemical withanolides from pichuberries can help prevent inflammation, linking them to pain relief and managing inflammatory diseases such as arthritis. They also display other significant benefits, including antimicrobial, antitumor, anti-inflammatory, and antibacterial effects.

Per Serving: Kcal 130.5, Protein 3g, Carb 22g, Fat 4g, Sodium 359mg, Dietary Fiber 2.5g
Daily Values: Fiber 10%, Vit C 43%, Vit A 55%, Vit D 5 52%, Calcium 5%, Iron 7%

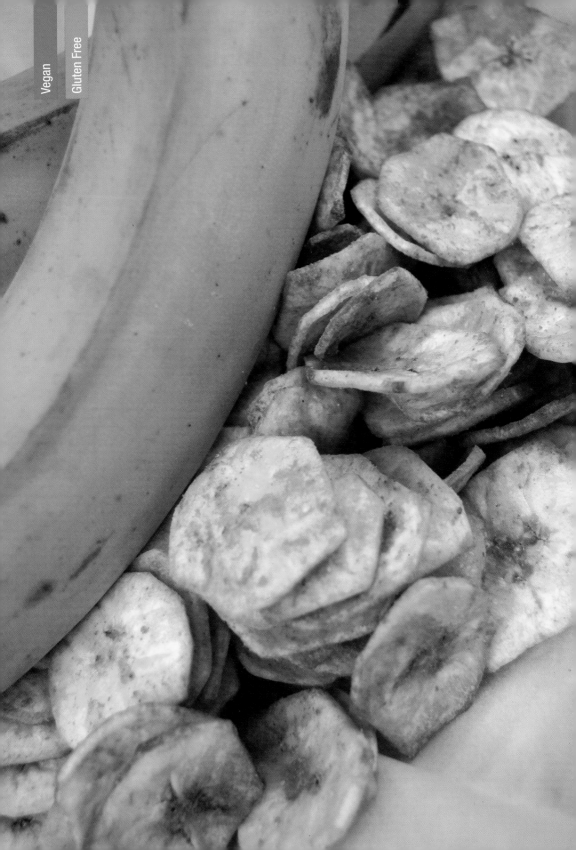

PLANTAIN CHIPS

Servings: 12 ♦ Serving size: ½ cup

Take a trip to the Amazon of Peru and experience the classic plantain chip, full of flavor without all the fat. We baked the chips instead of frying them and added spices for a complete belly-fat burn.

3 large green plantains

2 tablespoons canola oil

1 teaspoon ground paprika

½ teaspoon ground cumin

Salt

❶ Preheat the oven to 400 degrees F. Line two sheet pans with parchment paper.

❷ Using a very sharp knife, cut the ends off the plantains and slice each into three equal-length portions. Holding each portion on its axis, carefully slice off the outer peel and discard. Cut the plantain into ⅛-inch slices, taking the time to make the slices consistent.

❸ Put the plantain in a large bowl with the oil, paprika, cumin, and salt. Toss to evenly coat all the slices.

❹ Distribute the plantain slices among the sheet pans in a single layer. Bake for 15 to 20 minutes until crisp and golden but not burned. Eat while warm.

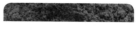

Paprika comes loaded with carotenoids—the pigments that give it its deep red color. It benefits your eyesight by preventing harmful light rays from damaging your eye tissues, while its vitamin A content aids in night vision.

Per Serving: Kcal 76.5, Protein 2g, Carb 4.5g, Fat 6g, Sodium 100mg, Dietary Fiber 0.5g
Daily Values: Fiber 2%, Vit C 3%, Vit A 4%, Vit D 5 0%, Calcium 0%, Iron 1%

POPPED KIWICHA

Serves: 1 ♦ Serving size: 1 cup

3 tablespoons kiwicha

Pop this grain into fluffy little kernels like micropopcorn. You can add it to multiple recipes or just eat it as a snack.

❶ Heat a medium frying pan over high heat until the entire surface of the pan is hot. Add 1 tablespoon of the kiwicha to the pan (no oil is needed); shake to distribute evenly across the surface. Cover the pan with a lid. Allow the kiwicha to "pop" and turn white in color, for roughly 30 seconds, making sure to shake the pan over the heat to avoid burning. When the kiwicha is popped, pour it into a medium bowl to cool.

❷ Repeat step 1 using the remaining 2 tablespoons of kiwicha. It may take a round or two of trial and error to get the heat, pan movement, and timing just right, but you will get the hang of it in no time.

NOTE: Store cooled, popped kiwicha in an airtight container at room temperature for one week.

Per Serving: Kcal 137, Protein 5g, Carb 24g, Fat 2.5g, Sodium 7.5mg, Dietary Fiber 3.5g
Daily Values: Fiber 14%, Vit C 3%, Vit A 0%, Vit D 5 0%, Calcium 6%, Iron 15%

POWER TRAIL MIX

Servings: 4 ♦ Serving size: ¼ cup

A perfect on-the-go snack between meetings, classes, or at the airport.

❶ Put all the ingredients in a small bowl and mix to combine. Store in an airtight container at room temperature for up to one month.

¼ cup cacao nibs

¼ cup dried pichuberries

¼ cup unsweetened coconut flakes

¼ cup roasted sacha inchi seeds *(or almonds)*

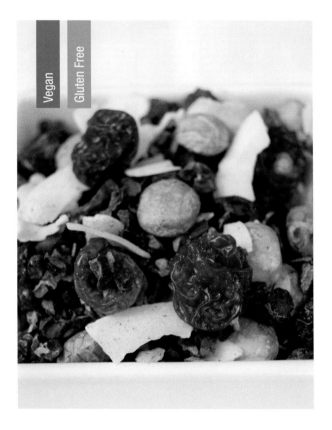

Vegan

Gluten Free

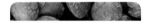

Sacha inchi seeds are loaded with protein at 9 grams per ounce, and rich in tryptophan, an amino acid that's a precursor to the production of serotonin, the important hormone that can help promote a positive mood.

Per Serving: Kcal 138, Protein 4g, Carb 6.5g, Fat 12g, Sodium 7mg, Dietary Fiber 4.5g
Daily Values: Fiber 18%, Vit C 2%, Vit A 3%, Vit D 5 3%, Calcium 1%, Iron 3%

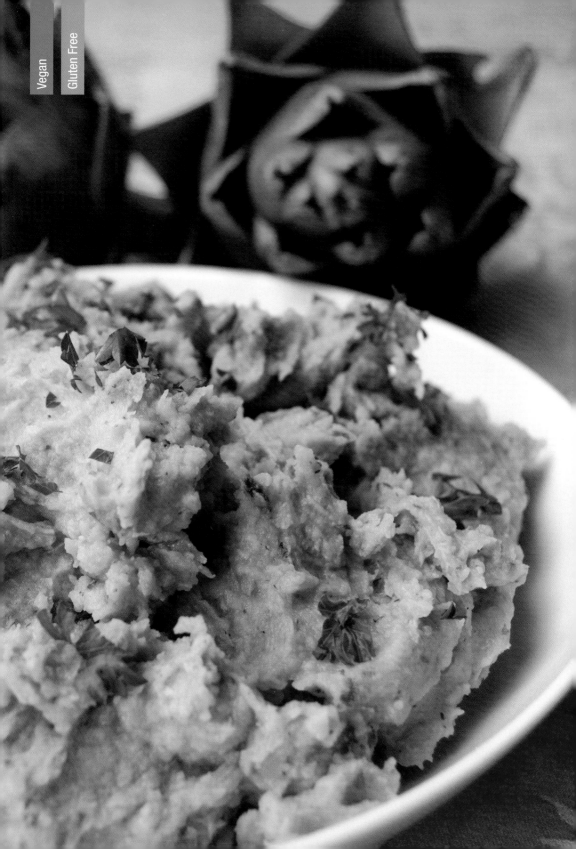

ROASTED ARTICHOKE MASHED POTATOES

Servings: 8 ◆ Serving size: 1 cup

Take your mashed potatoes to a level that is out-of-this-world astounding! Accompany your main dishes with this side on any normal night or amaze your guests at your next party.

3 pounds red potatoes, quartered

1 large red onion, diced into ½-inch pieces

2 cans *(14 ounces each)* artichoke hearts packed in water, drained

3 tablespoons olive oil

1 tablespoon dried oregano

1 tablespoon dried thyme

1½ cups chicken or vegetable stock

Salt and pepper

❶ Preheat the oven to 450 degrees F.

❷ Place the potatoes, onion, artichoke hearts, oil, oregano, and thyme on a large baking sheet or roasting pan. Toss the ingredients with your hands to evenly coat all the vegetables. Roast for 25 to 30 minutes until soft and fragrant.

❸ While the vegetables are still hot, carefully transfer them to a large saucepan. Add the stock and warm over medium heat. Using a potato masher, carefully mash the vegetables until they take on a light and fluffy texture. If the consistency is thicker than you like, add more stock. Add salt and pepper to taste.

Artichokes help protect liver cells. They contain silymarin, which is a flavonoid that supports liver health.

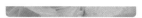

Per Serving: Kcal 260.5, Protein 4.5g, Carb 38g, Fat 13g, Sodium 650mg, Dietary Fiber 7g
Daily Values: Fiber 29%, Vit C 62%, Vit A 1%, Vit D 5 0%, Calcium 4%, Iron 13%

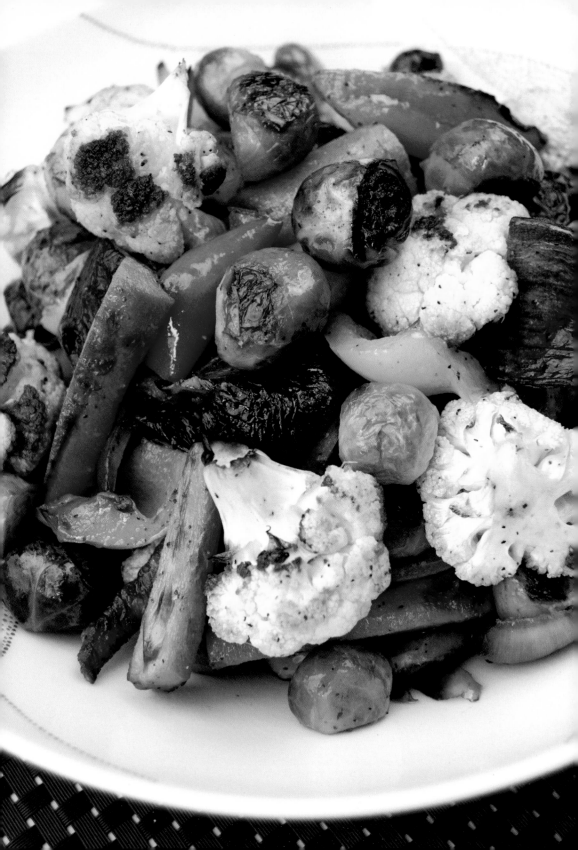

ROASTED VEGETABLES

Servings: 6 ◆ Serving size: 1 cup

This is a multicolored roasted vegetable recipe that you can add to soups, pastas, salads, and stews.

❶ Preheat the oven to 450 degrees F.

❷ Chop all the vegetables into pieces of equivalent size, about 1 to 2 inches in size.

❸ Put the chopped vegetables in a roasting pan with the oil and season with salt and pepper to taste. Toss to combine.

❹ Roast the vegetables for 20 minutes or until tender and the edges are browned.

1 medium red onion

1 medium bell pepper

1 medium zucchini

1 medium carrot

2 cups Brussels sprouts

1 head cauliflower, florets only

¼ cup olive oil

Salt and pepper

Per Serving: Kcal 140.5, Protein 4g, Carb 13g, Fat 9.5g, Sodium 50mg, Dietary Fiber 5g
Daily Values: Fiber 20%, Vit C 160%, Vit A 40%, Vit D 5 0%, Calcium 5%, Iron 7%

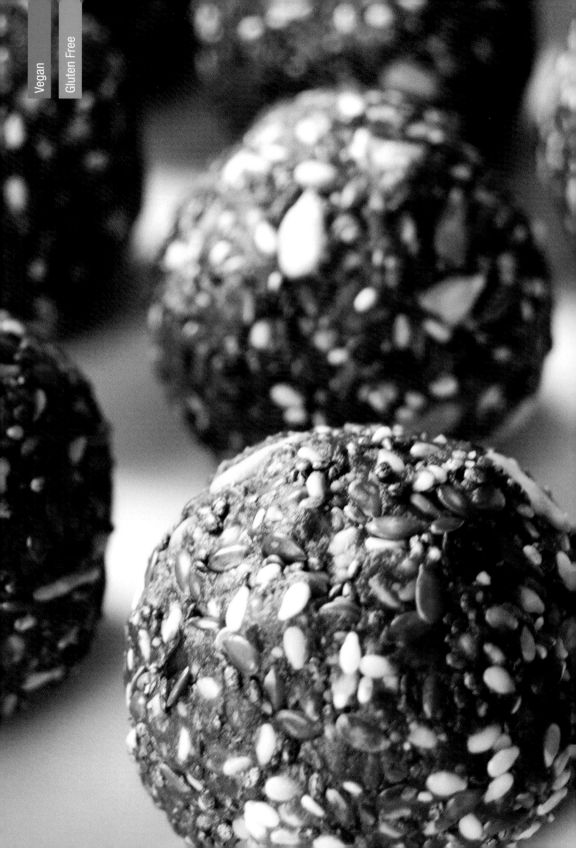

SUPERFOOD FOUR-SEED BITES

Servings: 20 ♦ Serving size: 1 bite

Enjoy this no-bake powerball. Boost your energy either before your workout or during your 3:00 PM midafternoon slump.

❶ Put the sesame seeds, chia seeds, flaxseeds, and sunflower seeds in a medium bowl and mix to combine. Set aside.

❷ Put the almond meal, dates, peanut butter, cacao, lucuma, agave, and salt in the bowl of a food processor. Process the mixture until it's well combined and the dates are broken down into pieces.

❸ Transfer the date mixture into the bowl with the mixed seeds. Using your hands, knead the seeds into the date mixture to form a "dough."

❹ Divide the mixture into twenty portions and roll them into 1½-inch balls.

NOTE: The superfood bites can be stored in an airtight container at room temperature for up to one week or in the refrigerator for one month.

¼ cup sesame seeds

¼ cup chia seeds

¼ cup flaxseeds

¼ cup shelled sunflower seeds

¼ cup almond meal

½ cup pitted dates

½ cup smooth peanut butter *(no sugar added)*

¼ cup cacao powder

2 tablespoons lucuma powder

¼ cup agave syrup

Pinch of salt

Don't let the tiny appearance fool you; chia seeds are packed with a fully balanced blend of protein, healthy fats, carbohydrates, and fiber— making them the ultimate energy booster.

Per Serving: Kcal 120, Protein 4g, Carb 13g, Fat 7g, Sodium 60mg, Dietary Fiber 3g
Daily Values: Fiber 12%, Vit C 1%, Vit A 0%, Vit D 0%, Calcium 5%, Iron 6%

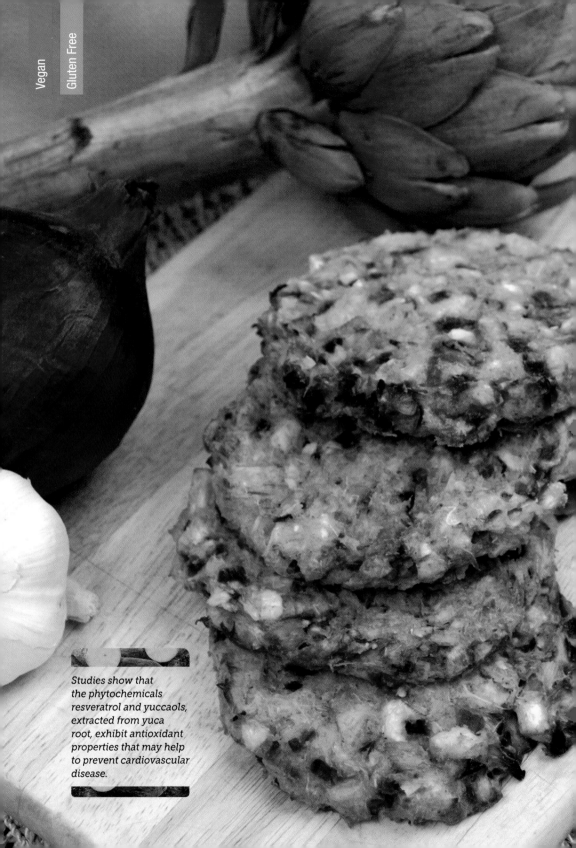

Studies show that the phytochemicals resveratrol and yuccaols, extracted from yuca root, exhibit antioxidant properties that may help to prevent cardiovascular disease.

YUCA ARTICHOKE PATTIES

Servings: 12 ♦ Serving size: One 4-inch patty

Yuca is normally deep-fried. This recipe mixes yuca with artichoke hearts to enhance the flavor, and it's baked, so you don't have all the added fat. Eat the patties over a salad or accompanied with grilled chicken or fish. You can even put your eggs on top of the patties instead of an English muffin for a faux eggs Benedict breakfast.

1 large yuca *(about 1½ pounds with skin on)*

Salt

1 can *(14 ounces)* artichoke hearts in water

1 tablespoon canola oil

1 medium red onion, chopped fine

4 cloves garlic, crushed

2 tablespoons ají amarillo paste *(or mild chili paste)*

2 teaspoons ground turmeric

Oil spray

1. Slice the yuca into three equal-length portions. Holding each portion on its axis, carefully slice off the outer peel and discard. Cut each portion in half lengthwise and chop into 1½-inch chunks.

2. Put the yuca in a medium-size saucepan and cover with water. Add the salt and place the pan over high heat. Bring to a boil, cover, and reduce to a simmer. Cook for 20 minutes or until the yuca is tender throughout. Drain and let cool.

3. Preheat the oven to 400 degrees F.

4. Drain the artichoke hearts, reserving the liquid. Dice the artichokes into ¼ to ½-inch pieces and set aside.

5. Put the yuca in a large bowl and mash it with a potato masher. Add the liquid from the artichoke hearts, ¼ cup at a time, to facilitate easier mashing. Set aside.

6. Heat the oil in a medium-size sauté pan over medium heat. When hot, add the onion. Once the onion starts to soften, add the garlic, ají, turmeric, and artichokes. Sauté until fragrant.

7. Add the sautéed mixture to the yuca and mix to combine. Season with salt to taste. Divide the mixture into twelve equal portions.

8. Spray two small sheet pans with a thin layer of oil. Flatten each portion of yuca into a 4-inch circle, about a ½ inch thick. Once all of the cakes are formed, spray them with a thin layer of oil.

9. Bake for 30 to 40 minutes until firm and golden.

Per Serving: Kcal 144, Protein 1g, Carb 32g, Fat 1.5g, Sodium 149mg, Dietary Fiber 1g
Daily Values: Fiber 3%, Vit C 3%, Vit A 0%, Vit D 5 0%, Calcium 2%, Iron 3%

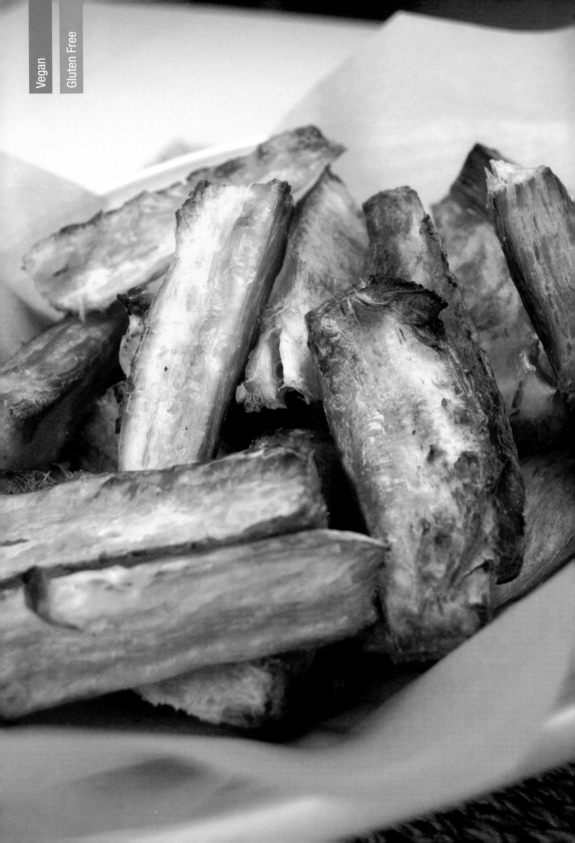

YUCA FRIES

Servings: 6 ◆ Serving size: 4 wedges

Yuca fries are a fantastic, healthy baked side dish to accompany any of your favorite meals.

1 large yuca *(about 1½ pounds with skin on)*

6 cups water

Salt

Coconut oil spray

❶ Slice the yuca into three equal-length portions. Holding each portion on its axis, carefully slice off the outer peel and discard. Chop each portion in half lengthwise and then into eight wedges.

❷ Put the yuca wedges, water, and salt in a medium saucepan over high heat. Bring to a boil, cover, and reduce to a simmer. Cook for 20 minutes until tender throughout. Drain and let cool.

❸ Preheat the oven to 400 degrees F.

❹ Place the cooled yuca on a large baking sheet and spray with coconut oil to coat. Season with salt.

❺ Bake for 40 to 50 minutes, flipping once halfway through the baking process, until the fries are golden in color. Serve warm that day.

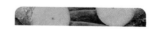

The yuca root has 3.7 grams of dietary fiber per one cup serving. Women need 25 grams per day and men should get 38 grams per day, according to the Institute of Medicine. Dietary fiber reduces the number of calories you consume by making you feel fuller faster and is therefore great for weight loss.

Per Serving: Kcal 60.5, Protein 0.5g, Carb 14g, Fat 0g, Sodium 0mg, Dietary Fiber 0g
Daily Values: Fiber 0%, Vit C 0%, Vit A 0%, Vit D 5 0%, Calcium 1%, Iron 1%

ROASTED SWEET PLANTAINS

Servings: 6 ♦ Serving size: ½ plantain

Coconut oil spray

3 large yellow plantains
with lots of black spots
(the blacker the better),
peeled

Salt

*Plantains are a staple food in Peru, and this is a
basic way to prepare them using a lot less fat.
Enjoy plantains as a side dish with most meals.*

❶ Preheat the oven to 400 degrees F. Lightly spray
a small roasting pan with coconut oil.

❷ Place the peeled plantains in the roasting pan
1 inch apart. Spray the tops with a thin layer of
coconut oil, followed by salt to taste.

❸ Bake for 30 minutes, turning them after the first
15 minutes of baking. The plantains should be
soft and well browned. Eat warm.

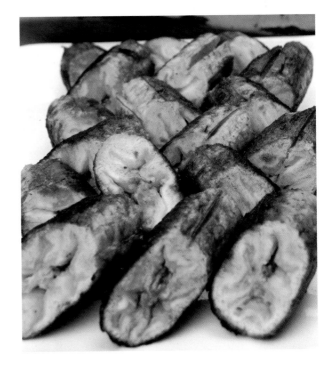

Per Serving: Kcal 112.5, Protein 1g, Carb 28.5g, Fat 1g, Sodium 3.5mg, Dietary Fiber 2g
Daily Values: Fiber 8%, Vit C 27%, Vit A 20%, Vit D 5 0%, Calcium 0%, Iron 3%

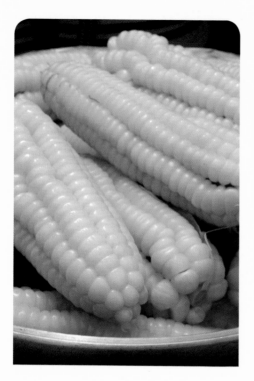
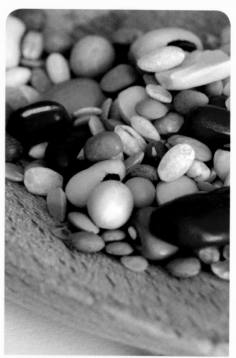

Staples

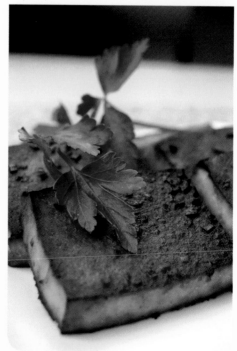

BOILED SWEET POTATO

Servings: 4 ♦ Serving size: ½ sweet potato

Boiled sweet potatoes are used as a side in many Peruvian dishes. You may also add them to salads, vegetables, protein dishes, and more.

2 large sweet potatoes

❶ Wash the sweet potatoes and put them in a medium-size saucepan, filling with water to cover. Bring the water to a boil over high heat, then lower the heat and cook at a simmer, covered, until the sweet potatoes are tender. Drain and let them cool slightly before eating.

NOTE: Sweet potatoes will keep in the refrigerator for three to five days.

Per Serving: Kcal 56, Protein 1g, Carb 13g, Fat 0g, Sodium 36mg, Dietary Fiber 2g
Daily Values: Fiber 8%, Vit C 3%, Vit A 184%, Vit D 5 0%, Calcium 2%, Iron 2%

CANNELLINI BEANS

Servings: 4 ♦ Serving size: 1½ cups

This is a classic recipe for cooking dry beans from scratch. It's not as hard as you think. You can cook most varieties of dried beans using this technique, too.

1 pound cannellini beans

4 cups stock (*vegetable, chicken, or beef*)

Salt and pepper to taste

❶ Put the beans in a stockpot and cover them with 3 inches of water. Let them soak for 4 hours. Drain the beans in a colander, discarding the water.

❷ Transfer the beans back to the stockpot and cover with 3 inches of water. Bring to a boil over medium heat. Drain the beans in a colander, discarding the water. This process helps remove the oxalates in beans, which are responsible for gastrointestinal discomfort.

❸ Transfer the beans back to the stockpot and add the stock. Season the beans with salt and pepper to taste. Cover, reduce heat, and cook the beans at a simmer for about 1 hour or until they are soft. Serve warm.

Per Serving: Kcal 392.5, Protein 26.5g, Carb 71.5g, Fat 1g, Sodium 158mg, Dietary Fiber 18g
Daily Values: Fiber 73%, Vit C 0%, Vit A 0%, Vit D 5 0%, Calcium 29%, Iron 68%

CHOCLO (LARGE CORN)

Servings: 4 ♦ Serving size: 1 cup

Choclo is the classic Peruvian corn that originated in the Andes. Traditionally, the large corn kernels are eaten with queso fresco and ají sauce for a quick and scrumptious snack.

1 pound frozen choclo desgranado

6 cups water

Salt

❶ Put the choclo and water in a medium saucepan over high heat. Bring to a boil, cover, and reduce to a simmer. Cook for 30 to 45 minutes until tender throughout. Drain and let cool.

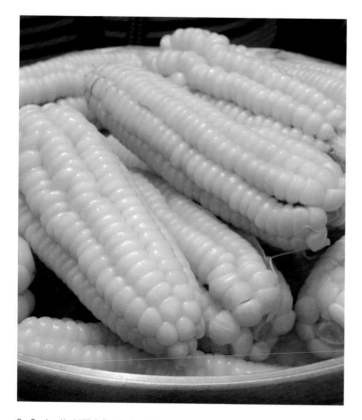

Per Serving: Kcal 157.5, Protein 4.5g, Carb 37.5g, Fat 0g, Sodium 22mg, Dietary Fiber 2g
Daily Values: Fiber 9%, Vit C 9%, Vit A 0%, Vit D 5 0%, Calcium 2%, Iron 13%

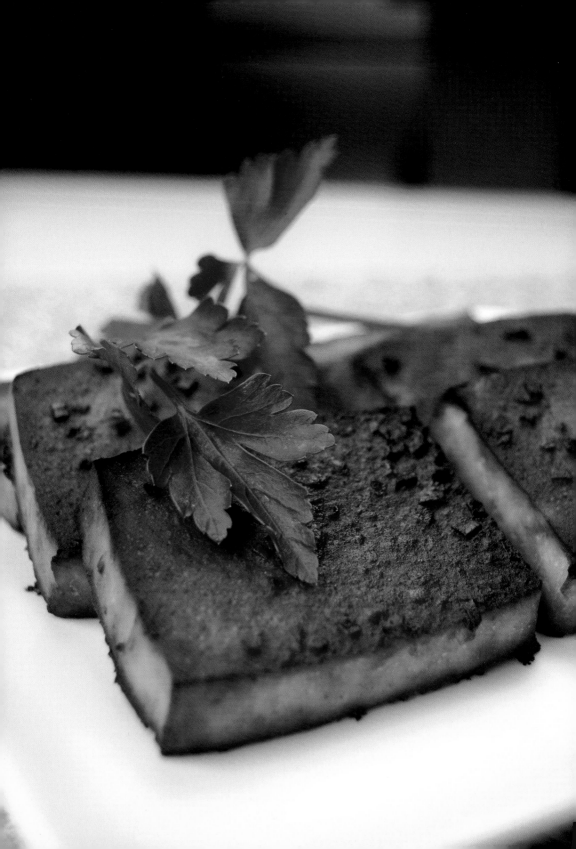

GARLIC ROASTED MISO TOFU

Prep the tofu on a weekend and use it throughout the week. Add to salads, grain dishes, vegetables dishes, or any dish where you want some extra protein.

Oil spray

1 tablespoon red miso

2 cloves garlic, crushed

2 tablespoons white vinegar

1 tablespoon Bragg's Liquid Aminos *(or low-sodium soy sauce)*

1 block *(14 ounces)* extra firm tofu, drained

❶ Preheat the oven to 400 degrees F. Lightly spray a small roasting pan with oil.

❷ To make the marinade, put the miso, garlic, vinegar, and Bragg's into a large, shallow bowl. Mix with a fork to create a smooth, homogeneous mixture. Set aside.

❸ Slice the tofu into six ½-inch slabs. Dip each piece of tofu in the marinade, making sure to coat all sides completely. Let the tofu rest in the marinade for 30 minutes (the tofu can also be left to marinate overnight in the refrigerator for convenience).

❹ Place each piece of tofu in the pan, ½-inch apart. Pour the remaining marinade over each piece of tofu.

❺ Bake for 30 minutes or until crisp and golden around the edges. Let the slices cool slightly before serving.

Per Serving: Kcal 81, Protein 7g, Carb 3.5g, Fat 4g, Sodium 231mg, Dietary Fiber 1g
Daily Values: Fiber 3%, Vit C 1%, Vit A 0%, Vit D 5 0%, Calcium 5%, Iron 7%

LENTILS

Servings: 4 ◆ Serving size: 1 cup

1 cup brown *or* green lentils

3 cups water

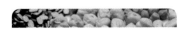

Lentils, a small but nutritional member of the legume family, are a good source of cholesterol-lowering fiber. Not only do lentils help lower cholesterol, they are of special benefit in managing blood-sugar disorders since their high fiber content prevents blood sugar levels from rising rapidly after a meal.

This is a basic way to cook lentils.

❶ Put the lentils in a sieve and rinse them under cold water until the water runs clear. Transfer them to a medium saucepan and add the water. Bring to a boil, cover, and reduce the heat to low. Simmer until all of the water has been absorbed, for 25 to 35 minutes.

NOTE: Lentils will keep in the refrigerator for three to five days.

Per Serving: Kcal 169.5, Protein 12.5g, Carb 29g, Fat 0.5g, Sodium 8mg, Dietary Fiber 14.5g
Daily Values: Fiber 59%, Vit C 4%, Vit A 0%, Vit D 5 0%, Calcium 3%, Iron 20%

QUINOA

Servings: 4 ◆ Serving size: 1 cup

1 cup quinoa, raw

2 cups water

A simple basic quinoa recipe.

❶ Place quinoa in a sieve and rinse under cold water until the water runs clear. Transfer to a medium sauce pot with 2 cups of water.

❷ Bring to a boil, cover, and reduce heat to low. Simmer until all of the water has been absorbed, for 15 to 20 minutes. Fluff with fork and serve.

NOTE: Quinoa will keep in the refrigerator for three to five days.

Per Serving: 222 kcal, Protein 8g, Carb 40g, Fat 3.5g, Sodium 13mg, Dietary Fiber 5g
Daily Values: Fiber 21%, Vit C 0%, Vit A 0%, Vit D 0%, Calcium 3%, Iron 15%

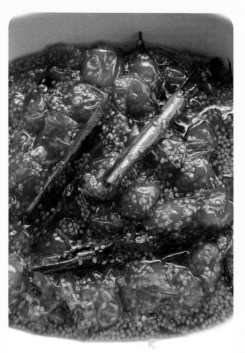

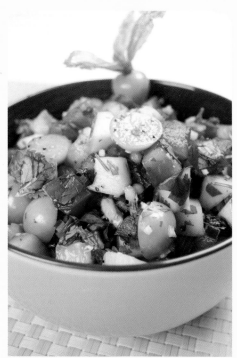

Dips & Condiments

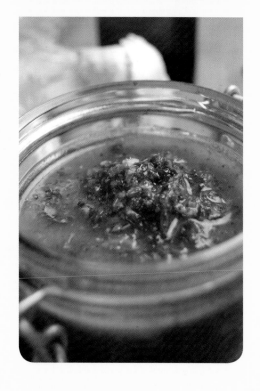

AJÍ VINAIGRETTE

Servings: 4 ◆ Serving size: 2 tablespoons

½ small red onion, chopped

2 tablespoons white wine vinegar

2 tablespoons ají amarillo paste *(or mild chili paste)*

1 tablespoon lime juice

1 tablespoon canola oil

Salt and pepper

This is great for adding to any salad or savory dish. Try it over causa and feel an extra tang of flavor.

❶ Put all the ingredients in the bowl of a food processor and process until smooth. Store in an airtight container, refrigerated, for one to three days.

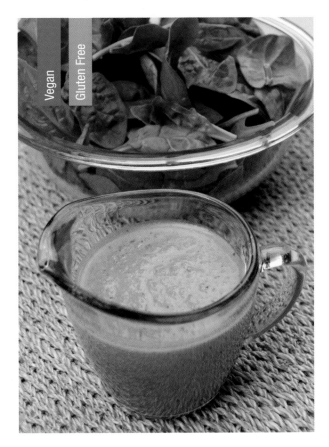

All across South America, peppers are a common ingredient in the local cuisine. The ají stands out as being exceptionally versatile since its characteristics are more fruity and smoky than spicy. It's great in sauces as well as incorporated with sautéed and grilled dishes.

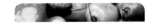

Per Serving: Kcal 42, Protein 0.5g, Carb 2g, Fat 0.5g, Sodium 1mg, Dietary Fiber 3g
Daily Values: Fiber 0%, Vit C 0%, Vit A 0%, Vit D 5 0%, Calcium 0%, Iron 0%

AVOCADO HUMMUS

Servings: 8 ◆ Serving size: ¼ cup

Hummus is a fabulous snack that can be made many different ways, not just with your typical garbanzo bean. Pair this creamy dip with your vegetable of choice.

❶ Put all the ingredients in the bowl of a food processor and process until smooth. Store in an airtight container, refrigerated, for one to three days.

1 can *(15 ounces)* garbanzo beans, drained

1 medium avocado, pitted and peeled

2 small cloves garlic, peeled

Juice of ½ lime *(about 1 tablespoon)*

¼ cup olive oil

¼ cup water

Salt and pepper

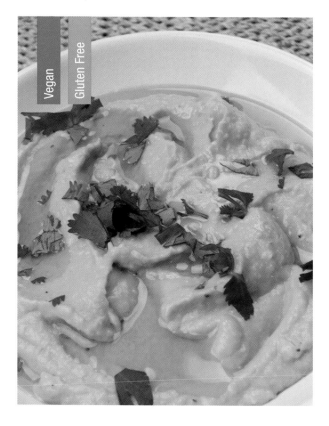

Vegan | Gluten Free

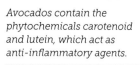

Avocados contain the phytochemicals carotenoid and lutein, which act as anti-inflammatory agents.

Per Serving: Kcal 131.5, Protein 2.5g, Carb 9g, Fat 10g, Sodium 183.5mg, Dietary Fiber 3g
Daily Values: Fiber 11%, Vit C 4%, Vit A 1%, Vit D 5 0%, Calcium 1%, Iron 3%

AVOCADO MANGO SALSA

Servings: 8 ♦ Serving size: ½ cup

1 mango, peeled and cut into ½-inch cubes

1 avocado, peeled and cut into ½-inch cubes

Juice of ½ lime *(about 1 tablespoon)*

1 tablespoon sacha inchi oil *(or olive oil)*

½ ají pepper *(or jalapeño)*, seeded and minced

2 tablespoons chopped cilantro

1 shallot, minced

Salt

Enjoy this salsa as a dip or over your protein of choice. Add salsa to your favorite entrées for extra flair.

❶ Put all the ingredients in a small bowl and mix to combine. Salsa will keep in the refrigerator for two to three days.

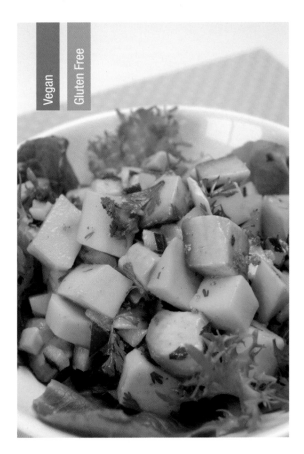

Vegan
Gluten Free

Sacha inchi oil is primarily composed of unsaturated fatty acids, mostly the omega-3 (alpha-linolenic) and omega-6 (alpha-linoleic) fatty acids. Omega-3 and omega-6 are considered essential because the body is unable to synthesize them. Consuming these fatty acids, primarily omega-3 fatty acids, can prevent diseases such as cancer, coronary heart disease, hypertension, and, potentially, rheumatoid arthritis.

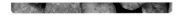

Per Serving: Kcal 64, Protein 0.5g, Carb 6.5g, Fat 4.5g, Sodium 5mg, Dietary Fiber 1.5g
Daily Values: Fiber 7%, Vit C 17%, Vit A 5%, Vit D 5 0%, Calcium 1%, Iron 1%

CHAMPAGNE VINAIGRETTE WITH PICHUBERRIES

Servings: 4 ◆ Serving size: 3 tablespoons

Because pichuberries are both tart and sweet, they're a perfect ingredient for salad dressings. Try this one over mixed greens with avocado or baked white fish like sea bass or cod.

❶ Put all the ingredients in a blender and process until smooth.

NOTE: This vinaigrette keeps well in an airtight container, refrigerated, for three to five days.

½ cup pichuberries

2 tablespoons champagne vinegar

1 tablespoon honey

1 tablespoon lemon juice

2 tablespoons sacha inchi oil *(or olive oil)*

Salt

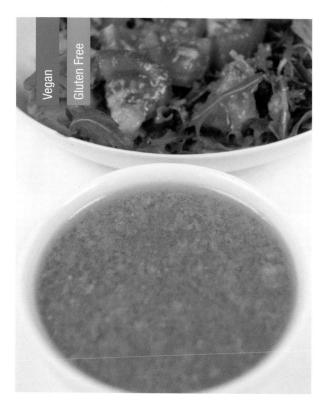

Vegan Gluten Free

Per Serving: Kcal 95, Protein 0.5g, Carb 7g, Fat 7g, Sodium 9mg, Dietary Fiber 0.5g
Daily Values: Fiber 1%, Vit C 6%, Vit A 6%, Vit D 5 7%, Calcium 0%, Iron 0%

CILANTRO CHIMICHURRI

Servings: 12 ♦ Serving size: 1 tablespoon

1 bunch cilantro,
roughly chopped

2 cloves garlic

2 teaspoons dried
oregano

2 tablespoons white
wine vinegar

½ cup sacha inchi oil
(or olive oil)

½ teaspoon salt

*An Argentinian-infused classic sauce using
sacha inchi oil to get your Peruvian powerhouse
on. Use this sauce over most proteins and meats,
as a salad dressing, or even drizzled over roasted
vegetables.*

❶ Put all the ingredients in the bowl of a food
processor and process until smooth and
homogeneous.

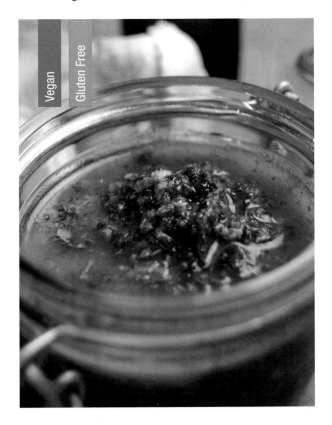

*By volume, sacha inchi
has more than 48 percent
omega-3s—that's more
than 84 percent of the
recommended daily value
of total essential fatty
acids. And those highly
concentrated omega-3s
fight disease-causing
inflammation.*

Per Serving: Kcal 89.5, Protein 0g, Carb 0.5g, Fat 9.5g, Sodium 98mg,
Dietary Fiber 0.5g
Daily Values: Fiber 1%, Vit C 1%, Vit A 2%, Vit D 5 0%, Calcium 1%, Iron 1%

CUCUMBER-CILANTRO LIME DRESSING

Servings: 4 ♦ Serving size: 2 tablespoons

Jamie Farnsworth, from the blog Girl Eats Greens (girleatsgreens.com), gave us one of her best vegan dressings, which tastes good on top of almost anything. Pour it on top of your favorite salad, protein of choice, or any grain, and you've got a ton of love in each bite.

❶ Put all the ingredients in the bowl of a food processor and blend until smooth. That's it! Add it to your favorite veggies, sandwiches, tacos, whatever you desire, and prepare to think twice about your everyday recipes.

2 cups chopped cilantro

2 tablespoons tahini

⅓ large cucumber

Juice of 1 medium lime *(about 1½ to 2 tablespoons)*

Salt

Vegan Gluten Free

Per Serving: Kcal 52.5, Protein 1.5g, Carb 3.5g, Fat 4g, Sodium 7mg, Dietary Fiber 1g
Daily Values: Fiber 3%, Vit C 10%, Vit A 12%, Vit D 5 0%, Calcium 2%, Iron 3%

Cilantro may be helpful for diabetics, as cilantro has been shown to lower blood sugar levels.

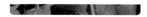

PICHUBERRY HONEY-MUSTARD DRESSING

Servings: 5 ◆ Serving size: ¼ cup

¾ cup low-fat Greek yogurt

2 tablespoons honey

2 tablespoons yellow mustard

½ cup pichuberries

This healthy dressing option can be added to your favorite spring salad mix or used as a dip for your crudités or chicken wings.

❶ Put all the ingredients in the bowl of a food processor and pulse until smooth and homogeneous.

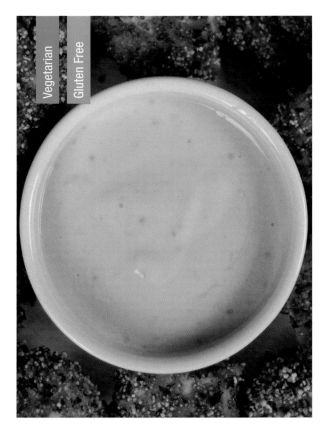

Per Serving: Kcal 64, Protein 4g, Carb 10.5g, Fat 1g, Sodium 89mg, Dietary Fiber 1g
Daily Values: Fiber 1%, Vit C 3%, Vit A 5%, Vit D 5 5%, Calcium 5%, Iron 1%

PICHUBERRY MARMALADE

Servings: 8 ♦ Serving size: 2 tablespoons

Here is another genius way to use the superfood pichuberry. This marmalade is a winner on top of waffles, cheese, crackers, ice cream, and more. This will be a hit at your next party, too.

2½ cups pichuberry halves

½ cup sugar

1 cinnamon stick

4 cloves

❶ Put all the ingredients in a small saucepan set over medium heat. Simmer for 25 to 30 minutes, stirring often, until the mixture thickens to a chutney-like consistency. Let cool to room temperature, then refrigerate in a sealed container for up to two weeks.

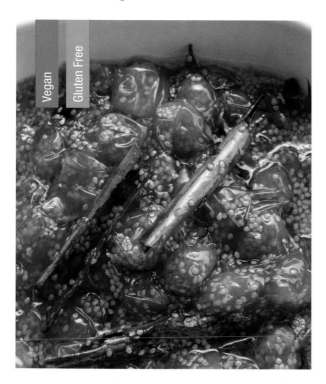

Per Serving: Kcal 77.5, Protein 1g, Carb 19g, Fat 0g, Sodium 21.5mg, Dietary Fiber 0.5g
Daily Values: Fiber 3%, Vit C 8%, Vit A 15%, Vit D 5 16%, Calcium 1%, Iron 0%

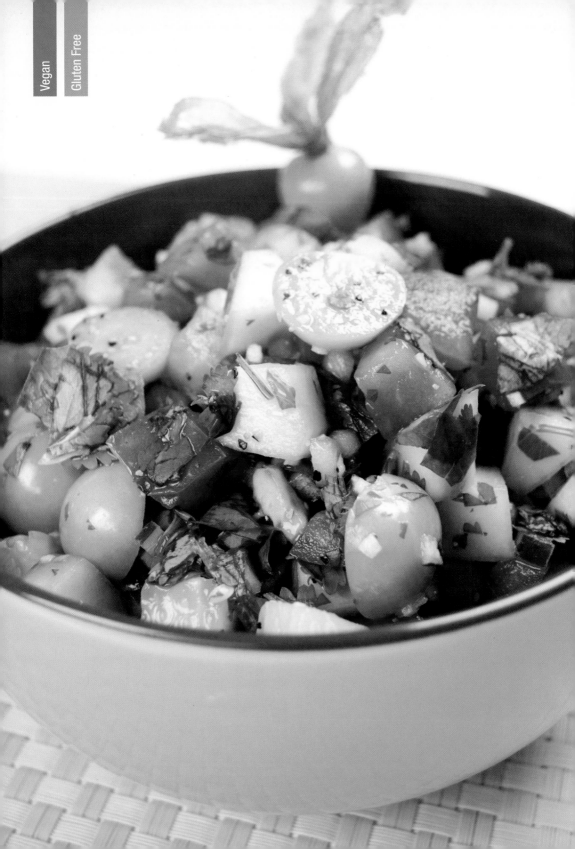

PICHUBERRY PICO DE GALLO

Servings: 8 ◆ Serving size: ½ cup

Who doesn't know pico de gallo? This salsa is Mexican-inspired and amazing when served over your favorite meat or grain dish. Add pico de gallo to almost every dish when you want to add some salsa. It's mouthwateringly delicious!

❶ Put the garlic, onion, vinegar, and lime juice in a small bowl. Mix and set aside for 15 minutes so the flavors can meld.

❷ Combine the pichuberries, cucumber, tomatoes, and cilantro in a large bowl. Mix in the marinated onion mixture. Toss to combine. Season with salt to taste.

1 clove garlic, minced

½ medium red onion, minced

1 tablespoon white wine vinegar

2 tablespoons lime juice

1 cup pichuberries, halved

1 medium cucumber, peeled and chopped into ½-inch cubes

2 large tomatoes, chopped into ½-inch cubes

1 cup chopped cilantro

Salt

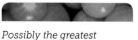

Possibly the greatest superfruit available in the United States, the pichuberry is a small orange fruit the size and shape of a cherry tomato.

Per Serving: Kcal 27.5, Protein 1g, Carb 6g, Fat 0g, Sodium 12mg, Dietary Fiber 1g
Daily Values: Fiber 4%, Vit C 15%, Vit A 15%, Vit D 5 7%, Calcium 1%, Iron 1%

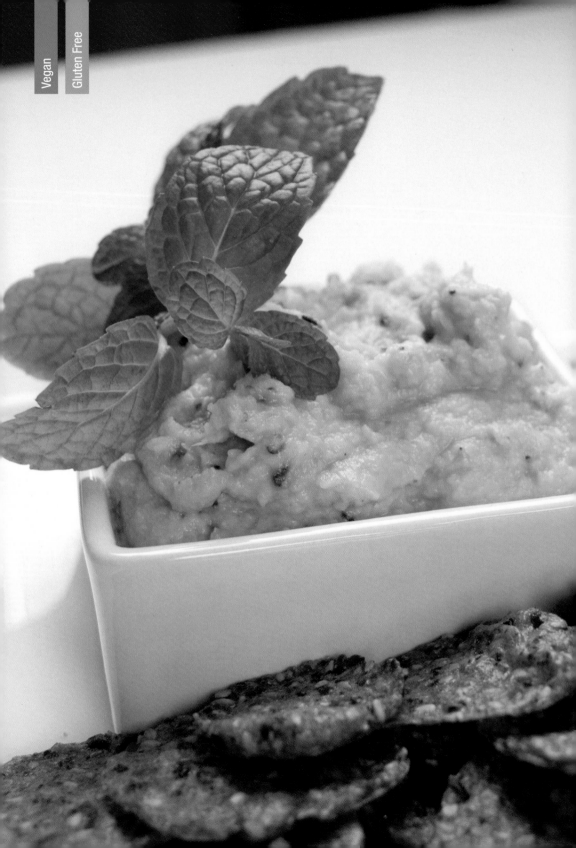

ROASTED GARLIC ARTICHOKE DIP

Servings: 4 ◆ Serving size: ¼ cup

This Mediterranean-inspired dip is a perfect snack with crackers or vegetables. Roasting the garlic enhances the flavor.

1 large head garlic

2 tablespoons olive oil

1 can *(15 ounces)* artichoke hearts in water, drained

½ teaspoon lemon juice

1 tablespoon sesame seeds

❶ Preheat the oven to 400 degrees F.

❷ Trim the top off the garlic head so that the flesh of each clove is exposed. Place the head on a sheet of aluminum foil and drizzle with 1 tablespoon of the oil. Wrap the garlic in the foil to seal. Bake for 45 minutes until soft. Cool slightly before using.

❸ Put the artichoke hearts in the bowl of a food processor. When the garlic has cooled, use your fingers to gently squeeze the garlic out of each clove skin. Add the garlic, remaining oil, lemon juice, and sesame seeds to the food processor and pulse the mixture until smooth.

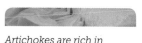

Artichokes are rich in vitamin C, calcium, fiber, and iron. They are low in both fat and calories.

Per Serving: Kcal 86.5, Protein 1g, Carb 3.5g, Fat 8g, Sodium 11.5mg, Dietary Fiber 0.5g
Daily Values: Fiber 2%, Vit C 6%, Vit A 0%, Vit D 5 0%, Calcium 4%, Iron 3%

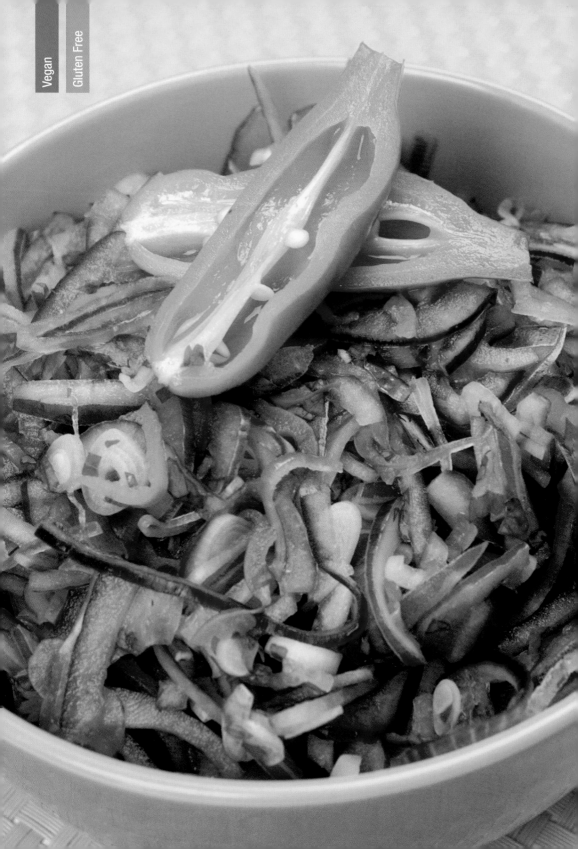

SALSA CRIOLLA

"Cebollita" is a term of endearment for onions. This is the most popular salsa in Peru and is used in sandwiches, rice, multiple proteins—you name it. This salsa may be added to most dishes.

❶ Peel the onions, slice them in half, and then slice them very thinly into half-moons. Put the onions in a large bowl with the salt. Cover them with cold water and let them rest for 10 minutes.

❷ Drain the onions in a colander and rinse with cold water to remove the excess salt. Lightly pat the onions with a paper towel to remove the water.

❸ Put the onions in a bowl with the peppers, lime juice, vinegar, cilantro, and salt and pepper to taste. Toss to combine.

NOTE: Salsa criolla is best the first day, but it will last in the refrigerator for three days.

2 medium red onions

1 tablespoon salt

2 ají amarillo peppers *(or jalapeños)*, seeded and slivered

¼ cup lime juice

2 tablespoons white vinegar

¼ cup chopped cilantro

Salt and pepper

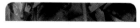

Cilantro has demonstrated both antibacterial and antifungal properties. In fact, some dental schools are studying how cilantro might be used for oral health.

Per Serving: Kcal 18, Protein 0.5g, Carb 3.5g, Fat 0g, Sodium 886mg, Dietary Fiber 0.5g
Daily Values: Fiber 2%, Vit C 7%, Vit A 1%, Vit D 5 0%, Calcium 1%, Iron 0%

ZESTY SACHA INCHI CILANTRO DRESSING

Servings: 4 ◆ Serving size: 6 tablespoons

3 cloves garlic

⅓ cup lime juice

2 tablespoons chopped cilantro

⅓ cup sacha inchi oil *(or olive oil)*

½ cup low-fat Greek yogurt

¼ teaspoon salt

¼ teaspoon pepper

Bursting with flavor, this dressing can be used over salads, vegetables, or as a dipping sauce.

❶ Put all the ingredients in the bowl of a food processor and pulse until smooth and homogeneous. Refrigerate for 15 minutes before serving.

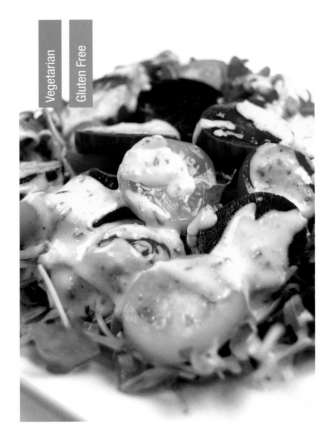

Vegetarian   Gluten Free

Some studies suggest that cilantro may improve sleep quality.

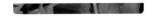

Per Serving: Kcal 202, Protein 3g, Carb 4g, Fat 19g, Sodium 158mg, Dietary Fiber 0.5g
Daily Values: Fiber 0%, Vit C 12%, Vit A 1%, Vit D 5 0%, Calcium 4%, Iron 1%

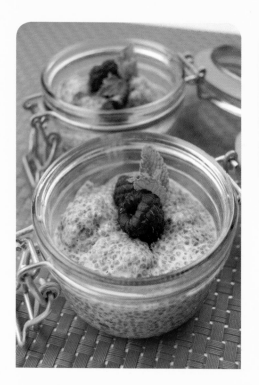

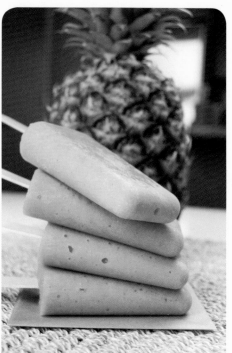

Sweet Treats

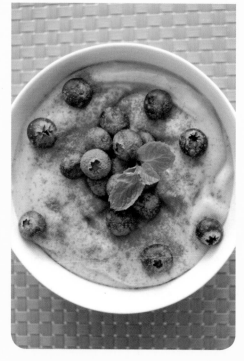

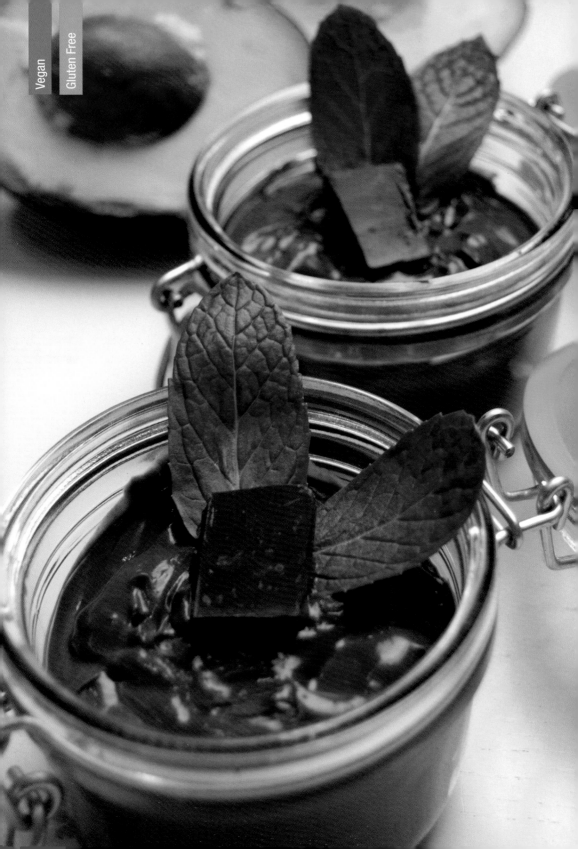

AVOCADO CACAO MOUSSE

Servings: 4 ◆ Serving size: ¼ cup

Calling all chocolate lovers! Silky, delicious, and anti-inflammatory, this mousse will rock your skin and your health.

1 ripe avocado
(without browning)

¼ cup cacao powder

3 tablespoons yacon syrup *(or agave syrup)*

¼ cup low-fat vanilla soy milk

Pinch of salt

❶ Scoop the flesh of the avocado into the bowl of a food processer. Add the cacao powder and yacon syrup and process until very smooth.

❷ Add the soy milk and salt to the mixture and process until smooth and homogeneous. Scrape down the sides using a rubber spatula and process one more time if necessary to obtain a pudding-like consistency.

❸ Chill the mousse for 1 hour before serving.

NOTE: This mousse is best eaten the day you prepare it.

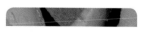

Avocados are packed with almost twenty essential nutrients, including fiber, vitamins B and E, folic acid, and potassium.

Per Serving: Kcal 104, Protein 2g, Carb 16g, Fat 6g, Sodium 163mg, Dietary Fiber 4g
Daily Values: Fiber 16%, Vit C 5%, Vit A 1%, Vit D 5 0%, Calcium 2%, Iron 5%

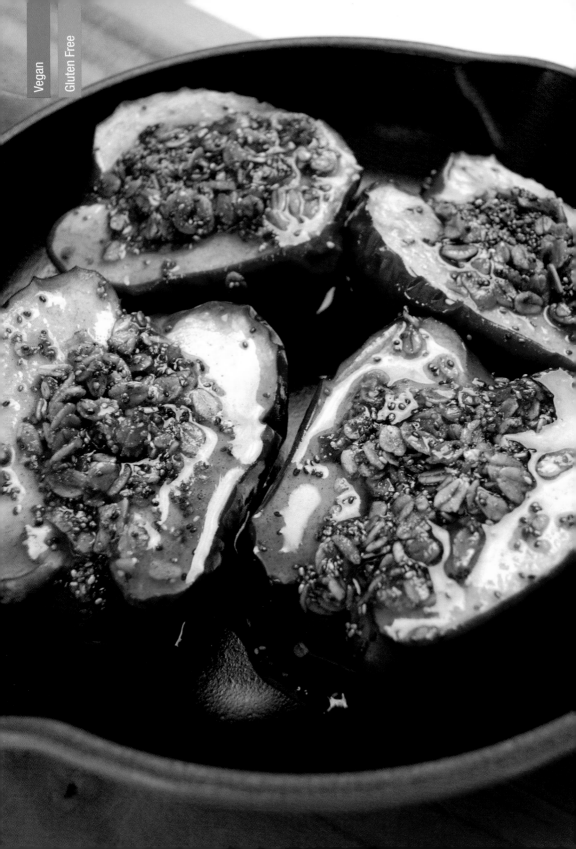

BAKED APPLES
WITH CINNAMON AND CHIA

Servings: 4 ♦ Serving size: ½ apple

This dessert is fast and effortless and perfect to make for a party or to just enjoy as an after-dinner treat. Your entire family will devour this fruity dessert.

❶ Preheat the oven to 350 degrees F. Lightly coat a small casserole dish with oil spray.

❷ Cut the apples in half. Remove the core and seeds using a melon baller.

❸ Place the apple halves in the casserole dish, cut side up. Bake, uncovered, for 15 minutes.

❹ While the apples are baking, combine the coconut oil, agave, oats, chia seeds, and cinnamon in a small bowl.

❺ When 15 minutes have passed, remove the apples from the oven. Spoon the filling into the center of each apple, then place the apples back in the oven. Continue baking until the apples are tender, for 15 to 20 minutes longer.

NOTE: Baked apples will keep in the refrigerator for one to two days.

2 large apples

1 tablespoon coconut oil, melted

2 tablespoons agave syrup

2 tablespoons old-fashioned rolled oats

1 tablespoon chia seeds

1 teaspoon cinnamon

Oil spray

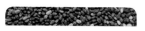

Chia seeds pack a powerful nutritional punch. They are a great source of fiber, calcium, manganese, magnesium, and phosphorus.

Per Serving: Kcal 126.5, Protein 1g, Carb 21.5g, Fat 5g, Sodium 1.5mg, Dietary Fiber 3.5g
Daily Values: Fiber 13%, Vit C 6%, Vit A 1%, Vit D 5 0%, Calcium 3%, Iron 3%

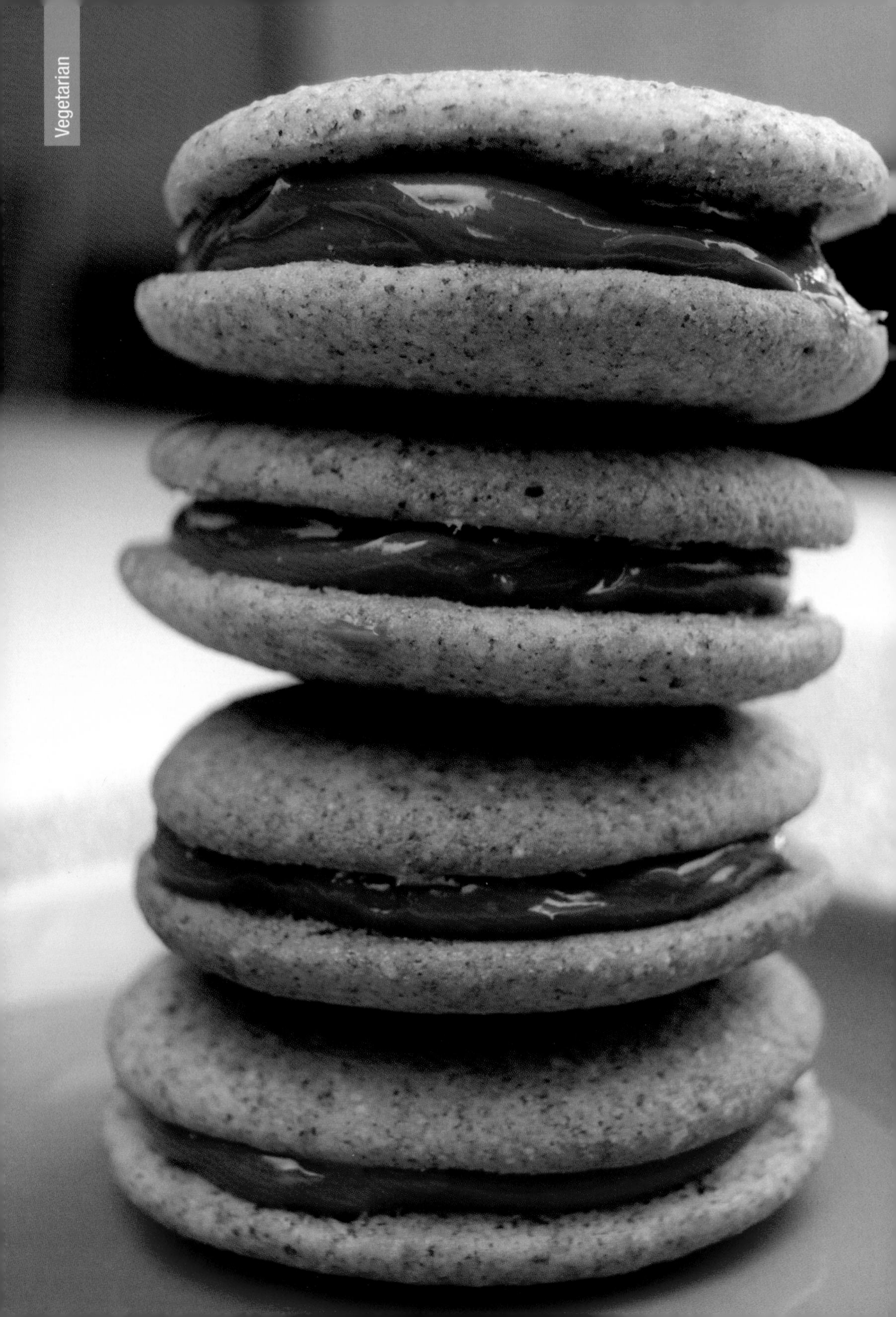

CAKEY BLUE CORN ALFAJORES

Servings: 16 ◆ Serving size: One 2-inch cookie

I have fond childhood memories of alfajores, a caramel or jam-filled cookie common to many parts of Latin America. We thank our friend and pastry chef, Chenoa Bol, for this variation on a classic. She paired the natural sweetness of blue corn meal with a dollop of dulce de leche, a rich and creamy caramel filling frequently used in Latin desserts.

¾ cup all-purpose flour

¾ cup blue corn meal

½ teaspoon salt

6 tablespoons unsalted butter, room temperature

½ cup granulated sugar

1 large egg, room temperature

1 tablespoon vanilla extract

½ cup low-fat milk

1 can *(13.4 ounces)* dulce de leche

❶ Preheat the oven to 350 degrees F. Line a baking sheet with parchment paper.

❷ In a medium-size bowl, whisk together the flour, corn meal, and salt. Set aside.

❸ Put the butter and sugar in the bowl of an electric mixer fitted with a paddle attachment. Cream the butter on medium speed until white and fluffy. Add the egg and vanilla and mix on low speed until combined. Scrape down the bowl with a spatula.

❹ Working in batches, add half of the flour mixture to the mixer and mix on low speed until just combined. Add ¼ cup of the milk and mix on low speed until just combined. Scrape down the bowl with a spatula. Repeat with the remaining flour mixture and milk.

❺ Using a tablespoon, drop level spoonfuls of batter onto the baking sheet, spaced about 2½ inches apart.

❻ Bake the cookies for 10 to 12 minutes or until lightly golden around the edges. Let them cool completely before moving on to the next step.

❼ Spread 1 tablespoon of dulce de leche on half of the cookies. Place the remaining cookies on top to form a sandwich.

NOTE: Will keep in a sealed container at room temperature for three days.

Per Serving: Kcal 172, Protein 3g, Carb 25.5g, Fat 6.5g, Sodium 81mg, Dietary Fiber 1g
Daily Values: Fiber 3%, Vit C 0%, Vit A 3%, Vit D 5 2%, Calcium 1%, Iron 2%

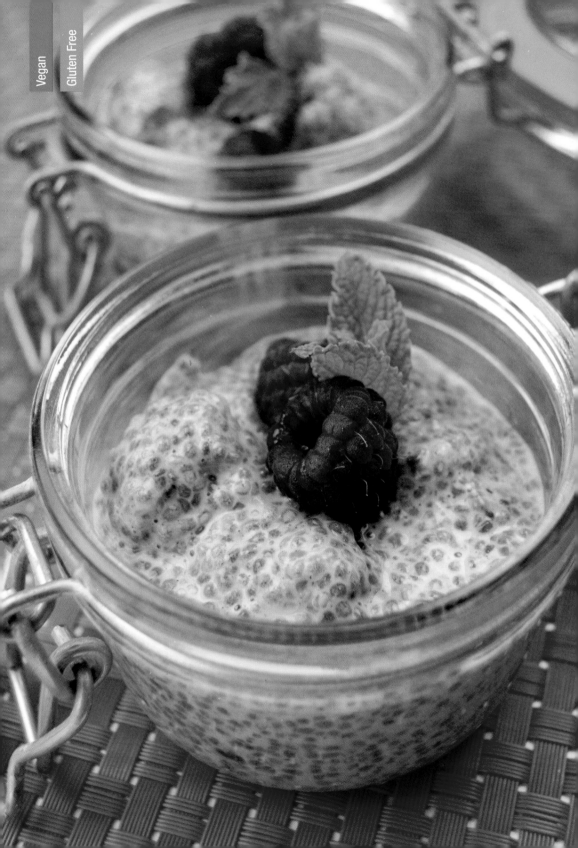

CITRUS RASPBERRY CHIA SEED PUDDING

Servings: 4 ◆ Serving size: ½ cup

This is super simple to prepare and it's vegan, too. The pudding is not extremely sweet, and it's very nice on the palate. Experience a light dessert to simply satisfy your sweet tooth.

❶ Put the almond milk, chia seeds, orange zest, and cinnamon in a small bowl and whisk to combine. Fold in the raspberries. Cover and refrigerate for 2 hours or until the texture is firm and pudding-like.

NOTE: The pudding will keep in the refrigerator for two to three days.

1 cup low-fat vanilla almond milk

3 tablespoons chia seeds

1 teaspoon orange zest

⅛ teaspoon ground cinnamon

1 cup raspberries

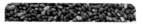

Chia seeds are high in omega-3 and omega-6 fatty acids, which help the body stabilize its blood sugar and slow down carbohydrate metabolism.

Per Serving: Kcal 71, Protein 2g, Carb 9.5g, Fat 3g, Sodium 37mg, Dietary Fiber 5g
Daily Values: Fiber 21%, Vit C 17%, Vit A 3%, Vit D 5 6%, Calcium 13%, Iron 6%

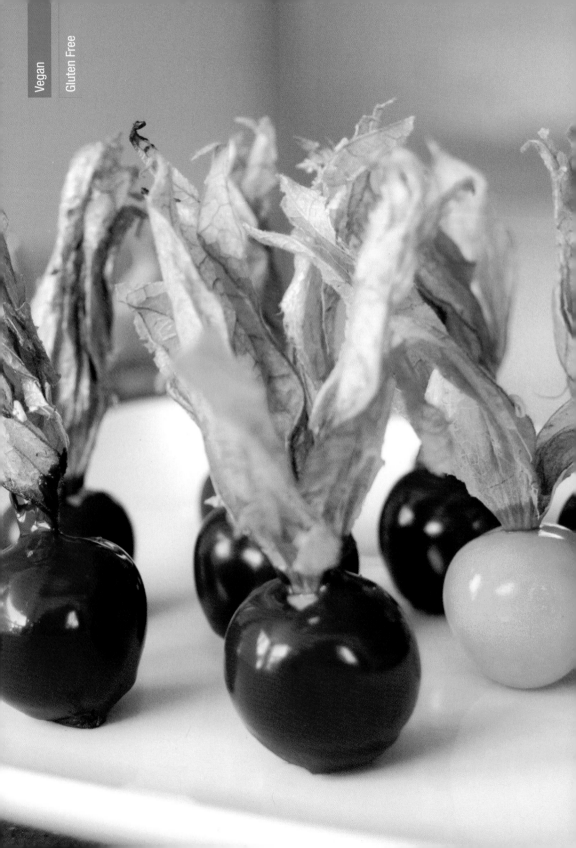

DARK CHOCOLATE–COVERED PICHUBERRIES

Servings: 12 ◆ Serving size: 1 pichuberry

A super low-fat and low-calorie dessert full of antioxidants—perfect for people who are trimming their waistlines while satisfying a sweet tooth.

½ bar *(50 grams)* **dark chocolate, 70–80%**

12 pichuberries

❶ Finely chop the chocolate and put it in a stainless steel bowl.

❷ Fill a small saucepan with 3 to 4 inches of water and bring to a boil. Place the bowl of chocolate so that it sits on top of the saucepan without touching the water. Lower the heat to a simmer and stir the chocolate until it's melted. Once melted, remove the bowl from the heat and stir until smooth and shiny.

❸ Dip each pichuberry, holding the husk out of the way, into the chocolate and cover completely. Place each pichuberry on a sheet of parchment paper or wax paper.

❹ Allow the chocolate-covered pichuberries to harden for about 30 minutes in the refrigerator.

NOTE: Store in the refrigerator for up to one week.

Pichuberries contain 1.7 grams of protein in just 3.5 ounces! And at just 65 calories, it's a diabetes- and weight-loss-friendly fruit.

Per Serving: Kcal 26, Protein 0.5g, Carb 2.5g, Fat 1.5g, Sodium 2.5mg, Dietary Fiber 0.5g
Daily Values: Fiber 2%, Vit C 1%, Vit A 2%, Vit D 5 2%, Calcium 0%, Iron 0%

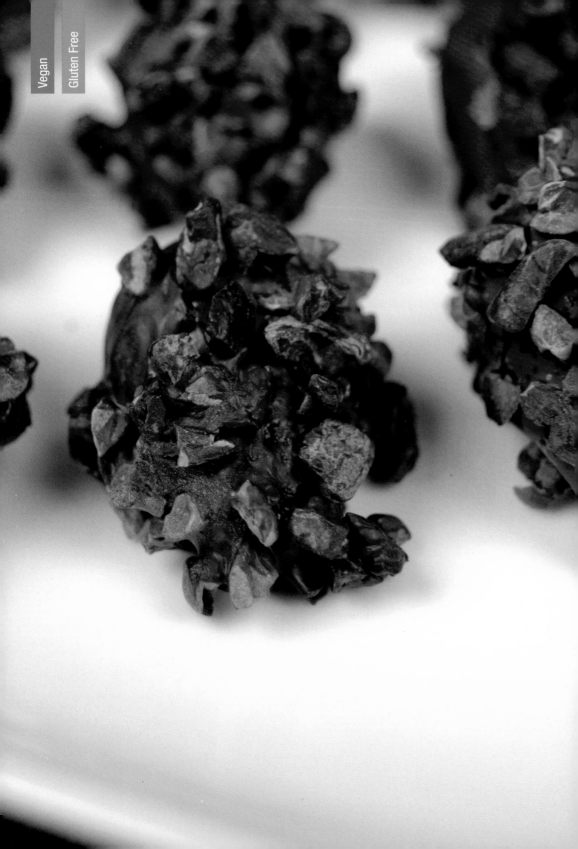

DARK CHOCOLATE FIGS
WITH CACAO NIBS

Servings: 12 ♦ Serving size: 1 fig

Chocolate lovers, get ready! You will be supersatisfied after just one of these guilt-free, delectable desserts.

½ bar *(50 grams)* dark chocolate, 70–80%

12 dried figs

½ cup cacao nibs

❶ Finely chop the chocolate and put it in a stainless steel bowl.

❷ Fill a small saucepan with 3 to 4 inches of water and bring to a boil. Place the bowl of chocolate so that it sits on top of the saucepan without touching the water. Lower the heat to a simmer and stir the chocolate until it's melted.

❸ Once melted, remove the bowl from the heat and stir until smooth and shiny.

❹ Dip the figs into the chocolate, covering the fig completely. Immediately roll the figs in the cacao nibs and place them on a sheet of parchment paper or wax paper.

❺ Allow the chocolate-covered figs to harden for about 30 minutes in the refrigerator.

NOTE: Will keep in the refrigerator for up to one week.

Cacao has more antioxidants than black tea, green tea, or red wine, which means it has the antioxidant power equivalent to vitamin C.

Per Serving: Kcal 66.5, Protein 1g, Carb 9g, Fat 4g, Sodium 1mg, Dietary Fiber 3g
Daily Values: Fiber 12%, Vit C 0%, Vit A 0%, Vit D 5 0%, Calcium 2%, Iron 2%

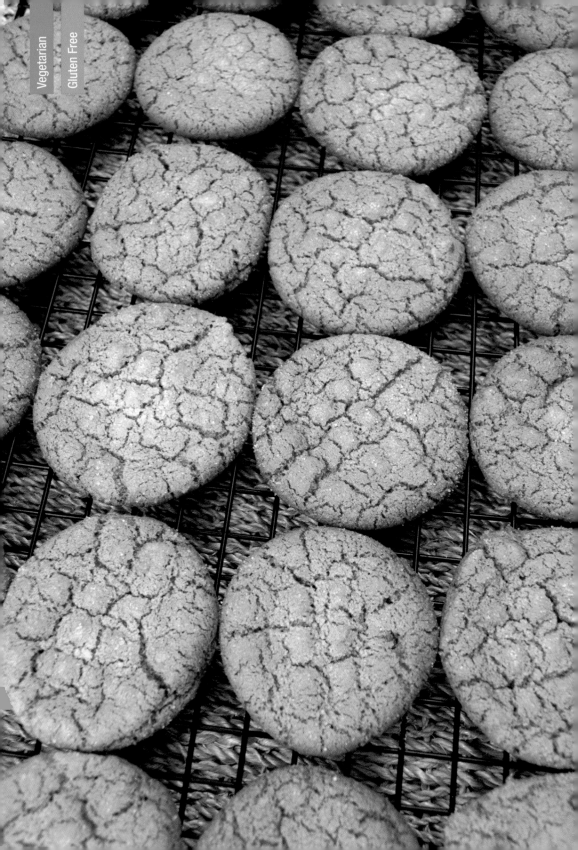

GLUTEN-FREE SACHA INCHI BUTTER COOKIES

Servings: 30 ♦ Serving size: One 2½-inch cookie

Everyone loves a butter cookie. Experience a Peruvian-inspired twist on the classic sweet recipe with the addition of omega-3s for brain health.

❶ Preheat the oven to 350 degrees F. Line a cookie sheet with parchment paper.

❷ Combine the egg, brown sugar, white sugar, vanilla, and sacha inchi butter in a large bowl. Whisk to combine.

❸ Add the oat flour, baking powder, baking soda, cinnamon, and salt to the bowl, and gently fold in with a rubber spatula until a smooth and homogeneous dough forms.

❹ Drop the dough by the tablespoonful onto the cookie sheet about 1 to 2 inches apart. Bake for 10 minutes or until set and lightly golden. Let the cookies cool before eating.

NOTE: The cookies keep well in an airtight container at room temperature for up to a week.

1 egg

⅓ cup packed dark brown sugar

½ cup granulated sugar

½ teaspoon vanilla extract

½ cup sacha inchi butter *(or almond butter)*

½ cup oat flour

½ teaspoon baking powder

1 teaspoon baking soda

¼ teaspoon ground cinnamon

Pinch of salt

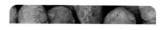

Sacha inchi has a high content of vitamin E. Vitamin E has been linked to a decreased risk for developing cardiovascular disease. Vitamin E is an antioxidant that helps fight free radicals, which can cause oxidative damage that leads to conditions such as cardiovascular disease.

Per Serving: Kcal 45, Protein 1g, Carb 6.5g, Fat 2g, Sodium 57mg, Dietary Fiber 0.5g
Daily Values: Fiber 2%, Vit C 0%, Vit A 0%, Vit D 5 0%, Calcium 0%, Iron 1%

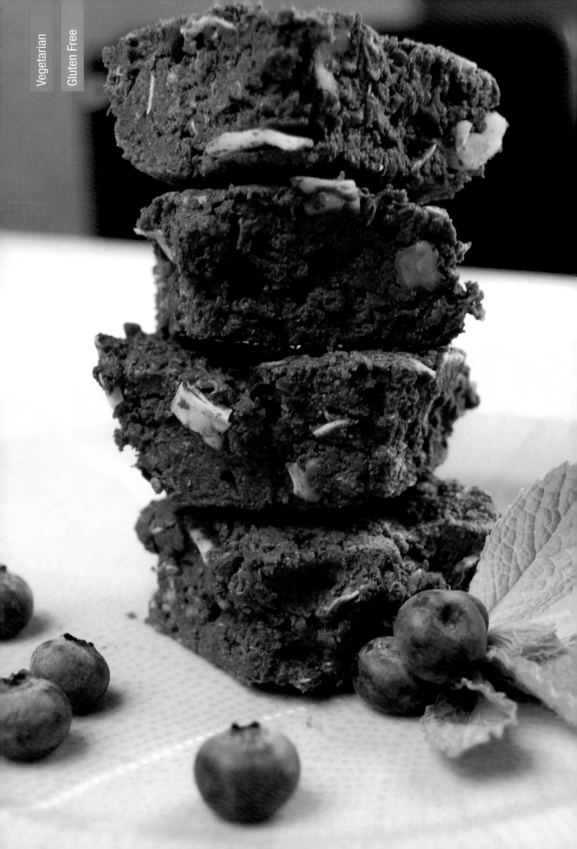

GLUTEN-FREE QUINOA FUDGE BROWNIES

Servings: 16 ♦ Serving size: One 2 × 2–inch square

While brownies are almost always served as a dessert item, this brownie uses quinoa flour, cooked quinoa, cacao powder, and coconut oil, easily doubling its use as an energy bar. Not only is it a great pre-exercise fuel, but it is also gluten-free.

❶ Preheat the oven to 350 degrees F. Coat an 8 × 8–inch square baking dish with coconut oil spray.

❷ Sift the flour, cacao powder, and salt into a large bowl and set aside.

❸ Put the coconut oil and the chocolate in a small microwave-safe bowl. Heat in the microwave for 30 seconds, remove, and stir. Heat for an additional 30 seconds, remove, and stir. The mixture should be completely melted. If it isn't, microwave it in 15-second increments, making sure not to burn it. Set aside.

❹ Whisk the agave, soymilk, vanilla, egg, and egg yolks in a medium bowl until combined. Add the melted chocolate and whisk until the liquids are well combined.

❺ Add the liquid mix to the flour mix and whisk until smooth. Fold in the quinoa, walnuts, and coconut until well incorporated.

❻ Pour the batter into the baking dish and put the dish in the oven. Bake for 15 minutes or until set. Once cool, cut into sixteen pieces.

NOTE: Store in an airtight container in the refrigerator for three to five days.

Per Serving: Kcal 155.5, Protein 4g, Carb 16g, Fat 8.5g, Sodium 49mg, Dietary Fiber 2.5g
Daily Values: Fiber 10%, Vit C 0%, Vit A 1%, Vit D 5 1%, Calcium 2%, Iron 6%

Coconut oil spray

1 cup quinoa or oat flour

½ cup cacao powder

¼ teaspoon salt

¼ cup coconut oil

2 ounces dark chocolate, chopped fine

¼ cup agave

⅓ cup vanilla soymilk

1 teaspoon vanilla extract

1 large egg

2 large egg yolks

1½ cups cooked quinoa *(see recipe on page 238)*

¼ cup chopped walnuts

¼ cup unsweetened shredded coconut

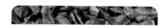

Cacao is rich in antioxidants, minerals, vitamins, and mood-enhancing nutrients called theobromine and phenylethylamine. The latter is a low-potency antidepressant that works like the body's dopamine and adrenaline. Phenylethylamine is known as the "pleasure chemical" because it's secreted by people in love.

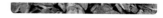

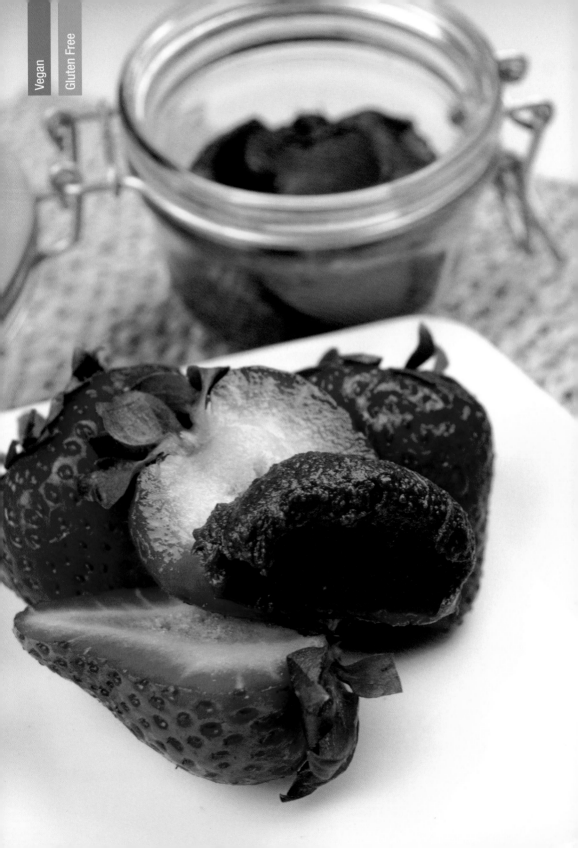

INCHI-TELLA

Servings: 7 ◆ Serving size: 1 tablespoon

For all you Nutella lovers out there, we have the perfect substitution—using protein-packed, omega-3-filled sacha inchi butter and antioxidant-friendly cacao powder. Enjoy your inchi-tella spread on a banana, or dip a strawberry in it.

❶ Put all the ingredients in a food processer and pulse until smooth. Scrape down the sides using a rubber spatula and pulse for 30 seconds longer.

NOTE: This spread keeps well in the refrigerator for about a week.

2 tablespoons sacha inchi butter *(or almond butter)*

2 tablespoons cacao powder

1 tablespoon agave syrup

5 teaspoons vanilla soy milk

Sachi inchi is a powerful antiaging food because it aids brain function, improves mental health and alertness, and boosts various brain functions like memory, intelligence, and thinking.

Per Serving: Kcal 55, Protein 2g, Carb 4.5g, Fat 3.5g, Sodium 13.5mg, Dietary Fiber 1g
Daily Values: Fiber 4%, Vit C 0%, Vit A 0%, Vit D 5 0%, Calcium 1%, Iron 1%

LUCUMA PUDDING

Servings: 4 ♦ Serving size: ½ cup

16 ounces *(1 block)* silken tofu

¼ cup lucuma powder

2 teaspoons vanilla extract

1 tablespoon agave syrup

Pinch of salt

Optional: Blueberries and cinnamon*

Lucuma has a maple-caramel flavor that enhances this silky, low-glycemic pudding.

❶ Put all the ingredients in the bowl of a food processer and pulse until smooth. Scrape down the sides using a rubber spatula and pulse for 30 seconds longer. Serve the pudding with blueberries and a sprinkle of cinnamon if desired.

NOTE: The pudding keeps in the refrigerator for three to five days.

*Cinnamon not included in the nutrient analysis.

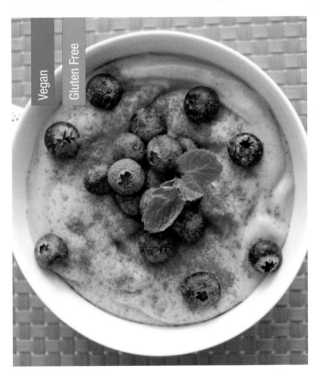

Vegan | Gluten Free

Lucuma is rich in antioxidants, fiber, minerals, and vitamins. It also has a good amount of beta-carotene, calcium, flavonoids, iron, magnesium, phosphorus, potassium, and vitamin B3, as well as fourteen essential trace elements.

Per Serving: Kcal 138, Protein 6g, Carb 18.5g, Fat 2.5g, Sodium 163mg, Dietary Fiber 0g
Daily Values: Fiber 0%, Vit C 0%, Vit A 0%, Vit D 5 0%, Calcium 3%, Iron 7%

PICHUBERRY PINEAPPLE SKEWERS

Servings: 4 ♦ Serving size: 1 skewer

This is a perfect snack for a sunny grilling day. Kids love to eat this finger-food snack for dessert, too.

Wooden skewers

2 cups pichuberries

1 can *(15 ounces)* pineapple chunks in juice, drained

DIRECTIONS:

❶ Place the wooden skewers in a casserole dish and fill with water to cover. Let them soak for 30 to 60 minutes before using.

❷ Prepare the skewers by placing the pichuberries and pineapple chunks, in an alternating pattern, onto the skewers.

❸ Heat up your grill according to the manufacturer's instructions. Grill the skewers, turning them as necessary, until they are lightly charred. Remove and eat warm or cold.

NOTE: The skewers are best if eaten the day of preparation.

Per Serving: Kcal 107, Protein 1.5g, Carb 26g, Fat 0g, Sodium 34.5mg,
Dietary Fiber 1.5g
Daily Values: Fiber 6%, Vit C 29%, Vit A 25%, Vit D 5 26%, Calcium 2%, Iron 2%

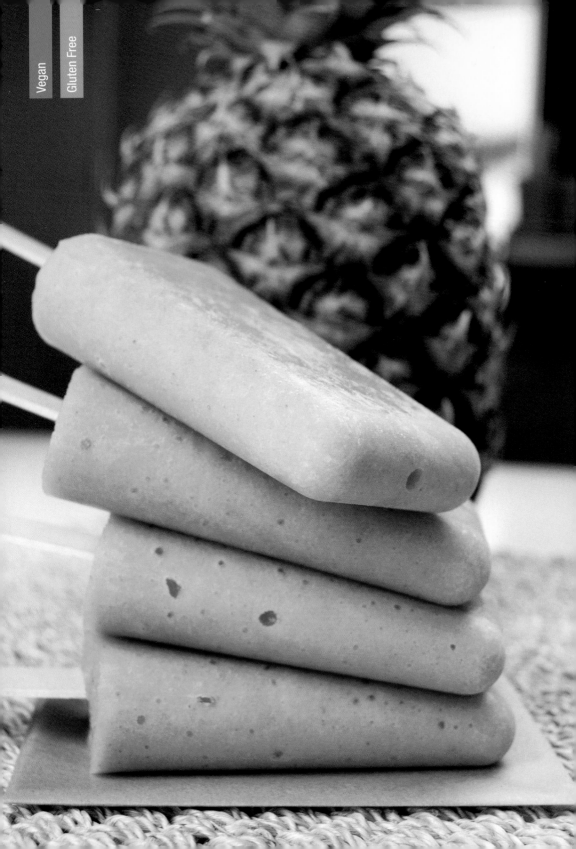

PINEAPPLE LUCUMA ICE POP

Servings: 6 ♦ Serving size: 1 ice pop

This sweet and refreshing fruit ice pop, made with low-glycemic lucuma and no added sugar, is perfect on a hot day or after a warm meal.

3 cups pineapple juice
(canned or prepared from 1 fresh pineapple)

½ cup lucuma powder

❶ If using a fresh pineapple, peel, core, and chop the pineapple into cubes. Puree enough of the pineapple to make 3 cups of juice. Save the remaining pineapple and eat it for dessert or blend it into smoothies.

❷ Put the juice and the lucuma in a blender and blend until smooth. Divide the mixture evenly among each ice pop mold.

❸ If you're using molds with attached sticks, place and secure the stick tops in the molds. If you're using freestanding sticks, freeze the ice pops for 30 minutes until slightly firm, then place the sticks in the center of each mold and finish freezing until they're solid throughout.

❹ To unmold the frozen ice pops, run them under warm water to loosen them from their molds.

NOTE: Ice pops will keep in the freezer for up to one month.

Per Serving: Kcal 146, Protein 2g, Carb 33.5g, Fat 0g, Sodium 9mg, Dietary Fiber 0.5g
Daily Values: Fiber 1%, Vit C 21%, Vit A 0%, Vit D 5 0%, Calcium 2%, Iron 5%

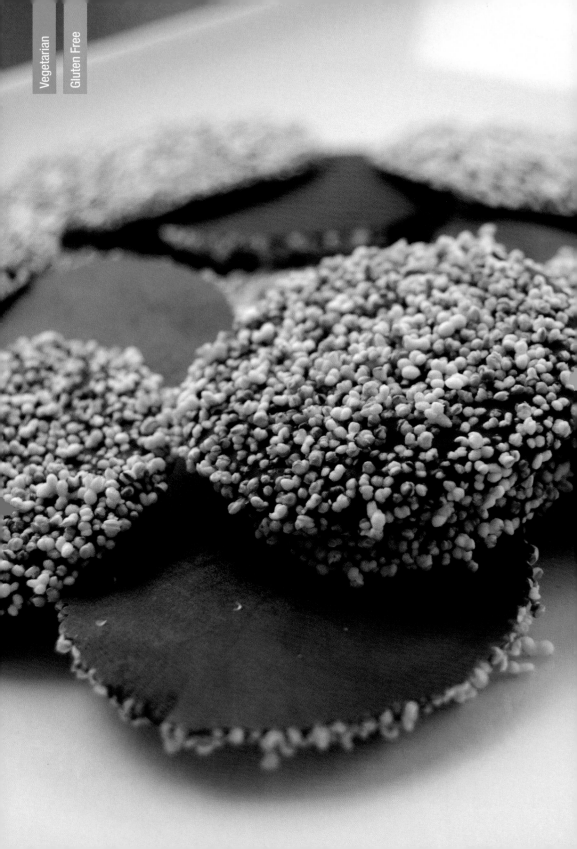

POPPED KIWICHA CHOCOLATE MEDALLIONS

Makes: 18 ♦ Serving size: 1 medallion

Are you a chocolate lover? We asked our friend and pastry chef, Chenoa Bol, how she would incorporate kiwicha into a dessert and she shared this simple yet sophisticated recipe. At only 30 calories per chocolate medallion, you can't go wrong!

1 bar 73% dark chocolate *(100g)*

½ cup popped kiwicha *(see recipe on page 220)*

❶ Finely chop the chocolate and put it in a stainless steel bowl.

❷ Fill a small saucepan with 3 to 4 inches of water and bring to a boil. Place the bowl of chocolate over the top of the saucepan without touching the water. Lower the heat to a simmer and stir the chocolate until it's melted. Once melted, remove the chocolate from the heat and stir until it's smooth and shiny.

❸ Place a piece of parchment paper on top of a baking sheet. Using a small metal spoon, pour small pools of melted chocolate onto the parchment paper, leaving some room for each medallion to spread out. Before the chocolate hardens, sprinkle each medallion with a generous layer of popped kiwicha.

❹ Allow the chocolate to harden for about 30 minutes in the refrigerator before eating.

NOTE: Will keep in the refrigerator for one to two weeks.

Per Serving: Kcal 34, Protein 0.5g, Carb 3g, Fat 2g, Sodium 0mg, Dietary Fiber 1g
Daily Values: Fiber 3%, Vit C 0%, Vit A 0%, Vit D 5 0%, Calcium 0%, Iron 0%

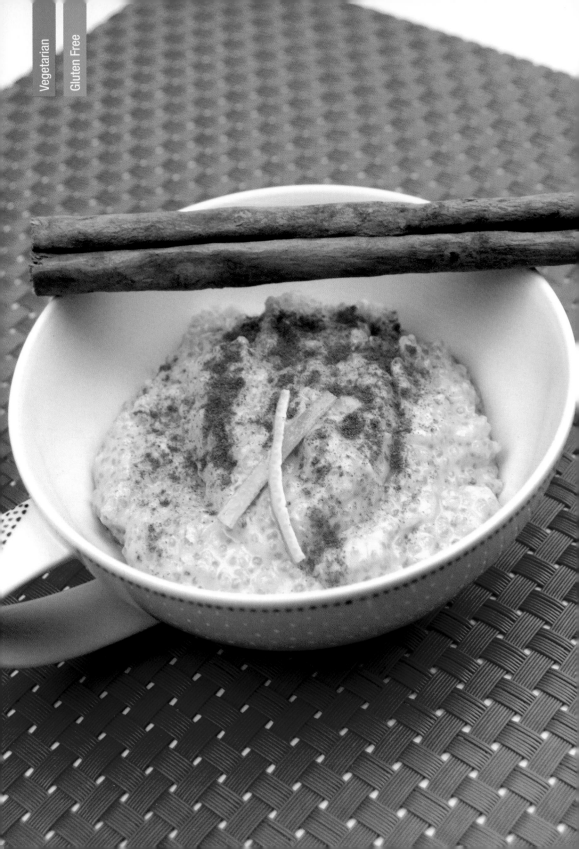

QUINOA CON LECHE

Servings: 8 ♦ Serving size: ½ cup

For this recipe, I used my abuela's (grandma's) famous recipe and added in extra protein and fiber by substituting quinoa for white rice. (Sorry, Abuela, I'm sharing the recipe with everyone!) This is one of my all-time favorite desserts. You will love this superfood version.

1 cup quinoa

3 cups low-fat milk

1 cup water

5 cloves

2 cinnamon sticks

1 teaspoon vanilla extract

Peel of 1 orange

1 can *(14 ounces)* sweetened condensed milk

❶ Put the quinoa, 2 cups of the milk, and the water, cloves, cinnamon, vanilla, and orange peel in a medium-size saucepan. Bring to a boil and then simmer, covered, over low heat until the quinoa is tender, for about 20 minutes.

❷ Remove the cloves, cinnamon sticks, and orange peel with a metal spoon and discard.

❸ Add the remaining milk and the sweetened condensed milk to the pot. Continue cooking over low heat, uncovered, until a pudding-like consistency is reached, for another 15 to 20 minutes. Stir the pot every few minutes, ensuring the pudding does not burn.

❹ Let the pudding cool to room temperature and then refrigerate until set. Enjoy cold.

NOTE: Quinoa con leche will keep in the refrigerator for up to five days.

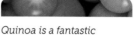

Quinoa is a fantastic source of fiber—a key nutrient needed for healthy blood-sugar regulation. It also provides outstanding protein quality, even in comparison to commonly eaten whole grains.

Per Serving: Kcal 283, Protein 10g, Carb 47.5g, Fat 6.5g, Sodium 109mg, Dietary Fiber 2g
Daily Values: Fiber 8%, Vit C 9%, Vit A 7%, Vit D 5 12%, Calcium 27%, Iron 12%

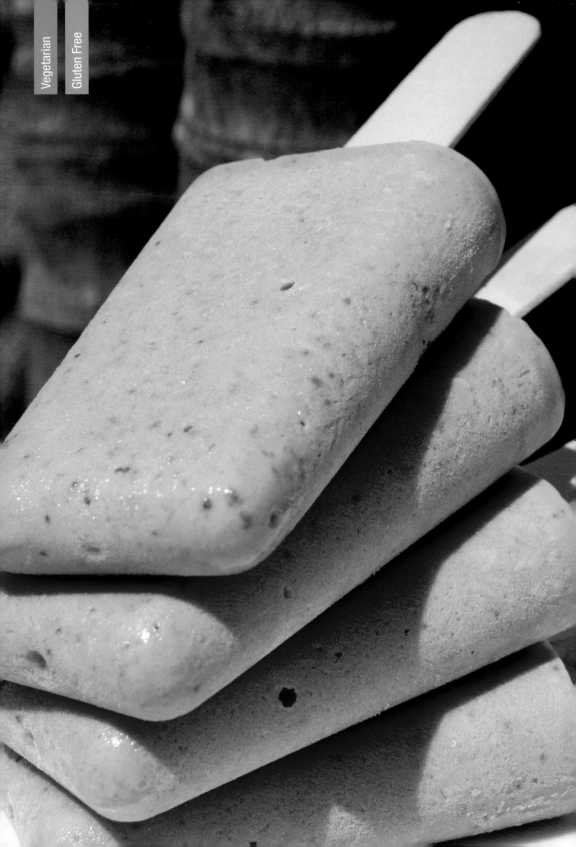

STRAWBERRY MACA FROZEN YOGURT POPS

Servings: 5 ♦ Serving size: 1 pop

Who says you can't have yogurt pops for breakfast? The strawberry maca frozen yogurt pop is the ultimate "start your day off right" combination: maca for increased energy and endurance, yogurt for bone and muscle health, and strawberries for immunity.

½ cup low-fat Greek yogurt

2 cups strawberries, fresh or frozen

2 tablespoons maca powder

2 tablespoons agave nectar

❶ Put all the ingredients in the bowl of a food processor and pulse until smooth. Divide the mixture evenly among each ice pop mold.

❷ If you're using molds with attached sticks, place and secure the stick tops in the molds. If you're using freestanding sticks, freeze the ice pops for 30 minutes or until slightly firm, then place the sticks in the center of each mold and finish freezing until they're solid throughout.

❸ To unmold the ice pops, run them under warm water to loosen them from their molds.

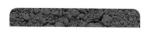

Maca may reduce anxiety and heighten sexual desire for both men and women. Studies suggest that by activating key endocrine glands, maca increases energy, vitality, and libido.

Per Serving: Kcal 75, Protein 3g, Carb 14.5g, Fat 0.5g, Sodium 10mg, Dietary Fiber 1.5g
Daily Values: Fiber 6%, Vit C 57%, Vit A 0%, Vit D 5 0%, Calcium 4%, Iron 2%

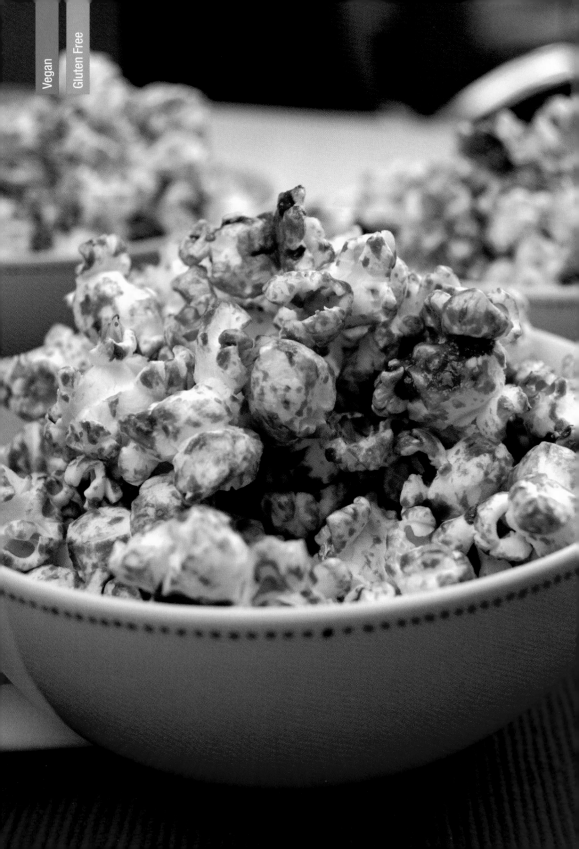

YACON "CARAMEL" CORN

Servings: 8 ◆ Serving size: 1 cup

I had the grand idea of making caramel popcorn using yacon. Now, every weekend, I make this recipe and watch a movie right in my own home. Friends and family who have visited me from Peru are now hooked on the popcorn, too. Get ready to become hooked on this amazing treat! (I like to prepare my popcorn using an air popper, per the manufacturer's directions, but if you don't have an air popper, you can pop it on the stove top.)

❶ Preheat the oven to 250 degrees F. Line a baking sheet with parchment paper.

❷ If you have an air popper, pop the popcorn according to the manufacturer's instructions. If you don't have an air popper, heat the coconut oil in a medium-size saucepan over high heat. Put four kernels in the pan and cover. When the kernels pop, add the remaining kernels. When the kernels begin to pop, gently shake the pan by moving it back and forth over the burner. Once the popping slows, transfer the popcorn to a heat-safe bowl. Return the pan to the stove top to pop any kernels that remain on the bottom.

❸ Heat the coconut oil, yacon syrup, and salt in a small saucepan over low heat. Whisk to combine. Once melted, drizzle over the popcorn and toss to coat.

❹ Spread the popcorn over the parchment-covered baking sheet. Bake for 10 to 15 minutes. Remove the popcorn from the oven and let it cool to room temperature. The popcorn should be crunchy and lightly sweet.

The nutritional analysis does not include the coconut oil.

Per Serving: Kcal 74.5, Protein 1.5g, Carb 12.5g, Fat 4g, Sodium 76mg, Dietary Fiber 2g
Daily Values: Fiber 8%, Vit C 0%, Vit A 0%, Vit D 5 0%, Calcium 0%, Iron 4%

½ cup corn kernels

2 tablespoons coconut oil *(if using the stovetop method to pop the corn)**

2 tablespoons coconut oil

2 tablespoons yacon syrup

¼ teaspoon salt

Yacon contains probiotics, the good bacteria that occur naturally in our intestines and keep bodily balance in check. Probiotics fight foreign invaders—or bad bacteria—in the gut.

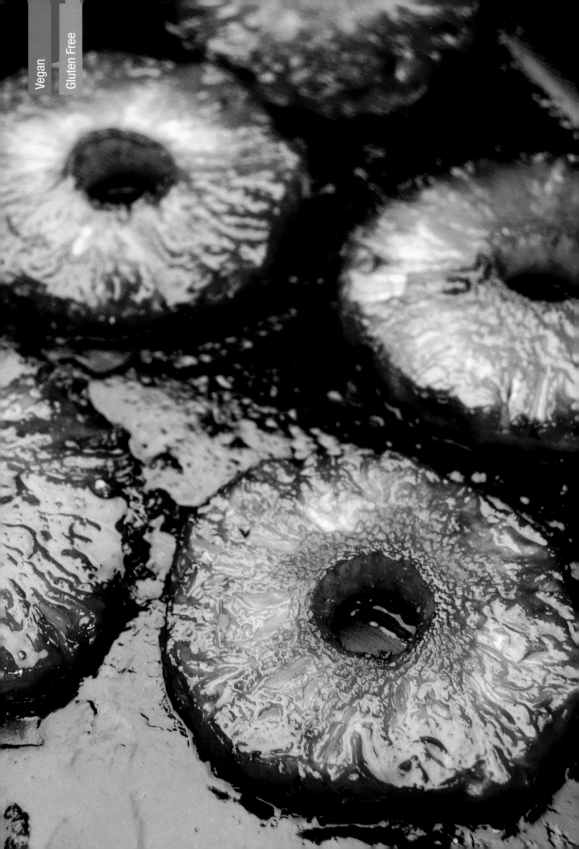

YACON ROASTED PINEAPPLE

Roasting pineapple brings out the sweet flavor of the fruit. By adding the yacon syrup, you get a caramelized, rewarding dessert. Put the pineapple on top of vanilla ice cream and be transported to heaven. Watch your portions!

Coconut oil spray

1 pineapple, peeled and sliced into ½-inch rounds

Salt

¼ cup yacon syrup *(or agave nectar)*

❶ Preheat the oven to 450 degrees F. Lightly coat a medium roasting pan with a thin layer of coconut oil.

❷ Remove the center core of each pineapple round using an apple corer or small round cookie cutter.

❸ Place the pineapple rounds in the roasting pan in a single layer. Spray the top of them with a thin layer of coconut oil, followed by a light sprinkling of salt. Drizzle with the yacon syrup.

❹ Bake for 20 minutes, flipping the slices halfway through. Eat that day served warm.

Per Serving: Kcal 41, Protein 0.5g, Carb 13g, Fat 0g, Sodium 79.5mg, Dietary Fiber 1g
Daily Values: Fiber 3%, Vit C 47%, Vit A 1%, Vit D 5 0%, Calcium 1%, Iron 1%

YUMMY STUFFED DATES WITH CACAO AND WALNUTS

Servings: 4 ♦ Serving size: 1 date

4 Medjool dates

4 teaspoons cacao nibs

4 whole walnuts

Walnuts and cacao are two of my favorite heart-healthy indulgences and both have been shown to help decrease inflammation. Combined with the dates, you've got a super-satisfying sweet tooth fix.

❶ Slice each date lengthwise so that the fruit forms a boatlike shape. Remove the pit and put 1 teaspoon of cacao nibs and a walnut inside each date.

NOTE: These are best eaten the day you make them.

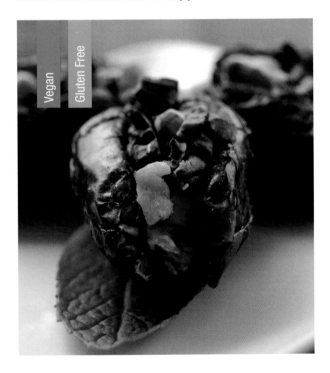

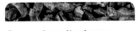

Cacao phenolics lower insulin resistance and sensitivity.

Per Serving: Kcal 112, Protein 2g, Carb 21g, Fat 4.5g, Sodium 0.5mg, Dietary Fiber 4g
Daily Values: Fiber 16%, Vit C 2%, Vit A 1%, Vit D 5 0%, Calcium 2%, Iron 3%

FRUITS & VEGETABLES
BY COLOR

Red	Blue/Purple	Yellow/Orange	White	Green
Beet	Blackberry	Acorn squash	Apple	Artichoke
Blood orange	Blueberry	Ají pepper	Banana	Arugula
Camu camu	Black currant	Apricot	Cauliflower	Asparagus
Cherry	Concord grape	Butternut	Cherimoya	Avocado
Cranberry	Eggplant	Squash	Date	Broccoli
Guava	Elderberry	Cantaloupe	Garlic	Broccoli rabe
Pink grapefruit	Mission fig	Carrot	Ginger	Brussels sprouts
Pomegranate	Plum	Golden kiwifruit	Jerusalem	Celery
Radicchio	Purple	Lemon	artichoke	Chayote squash
Radish	artichoke	Lucuma	Jicama	Chinese
Raspberry	Purple	Mango	Kohlrabi	cabbage
Red grape	asparagus	Nectarine	Mushroom	Cilantro
Red onion	Purple	Orange	Onion	Collard greens
Red pepper	cabbage	Papaya	Parsnip	Cucumber
Rhubarb	Purple carrot	Peach	Pear	Endive
Strawberry	Purple corn	Persimmon	Turnip	Green beans
Tomato	Purple endive	Pichuberry	White corn	Green grape
Watermelon	Purple peppers	Pineapple	White	Green peppers
	Purple	Plantain	nectarine	Honeydew
	potatoes	Pumpkin	White peach	Kale
	Shallot	Rutabaga	White potato	Kiwifruit
		Star fruit	Yuca	Leeks
		Sweet corn		Lettuce
		Sweet potato		Lime
		Tangerine		Okra
		Yellow beet		Peas
		Yellow		Scallions
		Grapefruit		Spinach
		Yellow pepper		Zucchini
		Yellow squash		

APPENDIX: WHERE TO FIND PERUVIAN SUPERFOODS

Ají: Ají, or "chili pepper" in the Peruvian regions of South America, has been a staple of Peruvian cuisine since the Incan Empire. Ají can be found in Latin markets or online at amazon.com and is sold pickled whole or as a chili paste. Ají amarillo corresponds to the fresh yellow pepper, while ají panca refers to the dried red pepper.

Artichokes: Produced in the United States and imported from many countries, artichokes are vegetables of the sunflower family. They are commonly found in mainstream supermarkets and farmers' markets while in season. Artichokes are a spring crop, with the tender artichoke heart tightly packed within layers of protective, semi-edible leaves. You can also find artichoke hearts packed in water in the canned foods section of most food markets.

Avocado: Largely produced in the United States, avocados are found in most supermarkets and in Latin and Asian specialty markets. They are available year-round and come in many different sizes and shapes depending on the variety. Haas avocados are most common to the United States.

Beans: High in protein and disease-fighting compounds, beans are a common staple food in the United States and around the world. There are many different sizes and types of beans, but all are of high nutritional value. Beans may be bought in raw, dried, or canned form and are found in food markets nationwide.

Cacao Powder and Nibs: This superfood was cultivated more than three thousand years ago by the Incans and has been labeled the "food of the gods." This magical food is now widely available in supermarkets, such as Whole Foods and Bristol Farms, and in your local supermarket as well as Latino markets. It can also be found online at eatingfree.com, navitasnaturals.com, and amazon.com.

Camu Camu Powder: Camu camu is a tropical fruit that varies between the size of a large grape and a small nectarine. Camu powder made from pulp is a convenient form that is available in specialty stores such as Whole Foods and Bristol Farms, and online at eatingfree.com, navitasnaturals.com, and amazon.com.

 Chia Seeds: Chia is a flowering plant of the mint family native to Mexico and Guatemala. The word "chia" is derived from the Nahuatl word *chian*, meaning oily, given that the plant's seeds are high in omega-3s. Chia seeds are growing in popularity in the United States and thus are available at all major supermarkets and online at eatingfree.com, navitasnaturals.com, and amazon .com.

 Choclo: Also referred to as Peruvian corn, choclo is a large and whitish corn kernel native to the Andes and is widely consumed in Central and South America, especially in Peru. Choclo is often described as chewier, nuttier, and less sweet compared to sweet yellow corn. Choclo can be found in Latin food markets.

 Cilantro: Growing in popularity throughout the United States, cilantro can be found in mainstream supermarkets as well as Latin and Asian grocery stores. Cilantro is often confused with Italian parsley at the market, but the citrusy aroma of cilantro can easily distinguish itself from the look-alikes.

 Kañiwa: Kañiwa is related to quinoa in its origin and use, in that it originates in the Andes of South America and was cultivated by the Incans as a key source of protein. Although quinoa is similar in shape and texture, the seeds of kañiwa are much smaller and boast a much darker pigment. Kañiwa is available at select supermarkets, in Latin food markets, and online at eatingfree .com and amazon.com.

 Kiwicha *or* Amaranth: Popularly known as amaranth, kiwicha is a "mini-quinoa" wonder grain in that it has an impressive amount of protein from concentrated amino acids. Kiwicha has been cultivated by people living in the Andes for more than four thousand years. It was a popular staple during the Incan Empire, but soon after it was abandoned in favor of other grains. Today, we are rediscovering the wonders of this tiny, health-packed seed that is now available at select supermarkets such Whole Foods, in Latin food markets, and online at eatingfree.com and amazon.com.

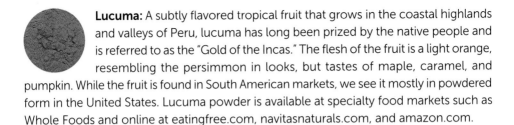

Lucuma: A subtly flavored tropical fruit that grows in the coastal highlands and valleys of Peru, lucuma has long been prized by the native people and is referred to as the "Gold of the Incas." The flesh of the fruit is a light orange, resembling the persimmon in looks, but tastes of maple, caramel, and pumpkin. While the fruit is found in South American markets, we see it mostly in powdered form in the United States. Lucuma powder is available at specialty food markets such as Whole Foods and online at eatingfree.com, navitasnaturals.com, and amazon.com.

Maca: This ancient Peruvian power food is prized for its ability to increase energy levels, improve endurance, and raise sexual drive and libido. A cruciferous vegetable, it is grown in Peru, dried, and then pulverized for easy use in shakes, cereals, and baked goods. Maca can be found in specialty stores such as Whole Foods and online at eatingfree.com, incaliving.com, sachavida.com, navitasnaturals.com, and amazon.com.

Papaya: Although considered an exotic fruit, papayas are readily available at mainstream supermarkets, as well as in Latin and Asian markets. They come in a variety of different sizes and colors depending on origin but carry the same overall nutritional value and health benefits.

Pichuberries: Pichuberries are possibly one of the greatest superfruits newly available in the United States at select stores such as Safeway, Vons, Bristol Farms, Whole Foods, HEB, Central Markets, Basket Market, Mollie Stone's Markets, Lucky Supermarkets, Save Mart, Stater Brothers, Publix, and Trader Joe's. Visit pichuberry.com to find a store near you or to make a purchase online. Though they originated in Peru, they are cultivated and imported by Colombia into the United States year-round.

Purple Corn: As with many of South America's abundant resources, purple corn almost became a lost crop, disregarded in favor of other grains and starches. Today, purple corn thrives in South America, as well as in American goods such as blue corn chips, tortillas, and cornbread. Purple corn can be found in specialty markets as well as Latin markets, and online at eatingfree.com and amazon.com.

Purple Potatoes: The distinct purple color in a purple potato distinguishes it from the more common yellow or russet potato. Originating in South America and imported to the United States, they are most commonly found as small spuds ranging from the size of a walnut to that of a Ping-Pong ball. Purple potatoes can be found at local supermarkets as well as Latin markets.

Quinoa: Imported from South America, and commonly used as a gluten-free substitute for rice and pasta, quinoa is widely available in most supermarkets and can be found in red, white, and black varieties.

Sacha Inchi Seeds & Oil: The sacha inchi plant produces star-shaped fruits with dark brown seeds inside that are the size of a macadamia. Despite the occasional reference to a "peanut," it is not a nut at all. In fact, it is a seed that can be eaten whole or pressed to extract its antioxidant-rich oil. Sacha inchi seeds can be found in some specialty markets such as Whole Foods, while both the seeds and oil are available online at eatingfree.com, incaliving.com, and amazon.com.

Sweet Potatoes: The pale purple skins and bright orange centers of sweet potatoes can easily distinguish them from other potatoes. They are readily found in supermarkets across the United States.

Yacon: Closely related to the sunflower, yacon is a crisp, sweet-tasting tuber that is traditionally grown and harvested in the northern and central Andes. Yacon can be found in the form of dried strips (similar to dried apple slices) or as a syrup and can be found online at eatingfree.com, navitasnaturals.com, and amazon.com.

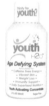

youthH2O: YouthH2O can be found online at http://www.youthh2o.com or in select locations such as GNC, Duane Reade, Vitamin World, HEB, Hy-Vee, the Vitamin Shoppe, Super Supplements, or online at drugstore.com, walgreens.com, and amazon.com.

Yuca: Also known as cassava, yuca is a shrub widely cultivated in South America for its starchy, tuberous root. Yuca is a major food staple for half a billion people around the world and can be found in the United States at farmers' markets, selective supermarkets such as Safeway and Whole Foods, and in Latin and Asian food markets.

SOURCES

Ají

Chan, Y. C., Chen, M. K., Lin, C. H., Lu, W. C., Wang, C. W. (2013). Capsaicin induces cell cycle arrest and apoptosis in human KB cancer cells. *BMC Complementary and Alternative Medicine* 13.

Derbyshire, E., Tiwari, B. K., Whiting, S. (2012). Capsaicinoids and capsinoids: A potential role for weight management? A systemic review of the evidence. *Appetite* 59:341–43.

Desmond, J., Kizaki, M., Koeffler, H., Kumagai, T., Lehmann, S., McBride, W., Mori, A., O'Kelly, J., Pervan, M. (2006). Capsaicin, a component of red peppers, inhibits the growth of androgen-independent, p53 mutant prostate cancer cells. *Cancer Research* 66:3222–29.

Artichoke

Anderson, J., Baird, P., Davis, R., Ferreri, S., Knudtson, M., Koraym, A., Waters, V., Williams, C. (2009). Health benefits of dietary fiber. *Nutrition Reviews* 67:188–205.

Di Venere, D., Fraioli, R., Linsalata, V., Miccadei, S., Mileo, A. M. (2012). Artichoke polyphenols induce apoptosis and decrease the invasive potential of the human breast cancer cell line MDA-MB231. *Journal of Cellular Physiology* 227, no. 9, 3301–9.

Florek, E., Horoszkiewicz, M., Kulza, M., Malinowska, K., Seńczuk-Przybylowska, M., Wachowiak, K., Woźniak, A. (2012). Artichoke—untapped potential of herbal medicine in the treatment of atherosclerosis and liver diseases. *Przeglad Lekarski* 69:1129–31.

Avocado

Byrns, R., Gao, K., Heber, D., Lee, R., Lu, Q., Wang, D., Wang, Y., Zhang, Y. (2010). California Hass avocado: Profiling of carotenoids, tocopherol, fatty acid, and fat content during maturation and from different growing areas. *Journal of Agricultural and Food Chemistry* 57:10408–13.

Chin, Y. W., D'Ambrosio, S. M., Ding, H., Kinghorn, A. D. (2007). Chemopreventive characteristics of avocado fruit. *Seminars in Cancer Biology* 17:386–94.

Domínguez, H., Juárez, C., Ledesma, L., Luna, H., Montalvo, C., Morán, L., Munari, F. (1996). Monounsaturated fatty acid (avocado) rich diet for mild hypercholesterolemia. *Archives of Medical Research* 27:519–23.

Hoffmann, G. & Schwingshackl, L. (2012). Monounsaturated fatty acids and risk of cardiovascular disease: Synopsis of the evidence available from systemic reviews and meta-analyses. *Nutrients* 4:1989–2007.

Beans

Anderson, J., Baird, P., Davis, R., Ferreri, S., Knudtson, M., Koraym, A., Waters, V., Williams, C. (2009). Health benefits of dietary fiber. *Nutrition Reviews* 67:188–205.

Arunasalam, K., Jiang, Y., Kakuda, Y., Mittal, G., Shi, J., Yeung, D. (2004). Saponins from edible legumes: Chemistry, processing, and health benefits. *Journal of Medicinal Food* 7, no. 1, 67–78.

Cacao

Andújar, M., Giner, R. M., Recio, M. C., Ríos, J. L. Cocoa polyphenols and their potential benefits for human health. (2012). *Oxidative Medicine and Cellular Longevity*, October 24, 2012.

Ismail, A. & Jalil, A. M. M. Polyphenols in cocoa and cocoa products: Is there a link between antioxidant properties and health? (2008). *Molecules* 13, no. 9, 2190–2219.

Camu Camu

Akachi, T., Kawagishi, H., Kawaguchi, T., Morita, T., Shiina, Y., Sugiyama, K. (2010). 1-methylmalate from camu-camu (*Myrciaria dubia*) suppressed D-galactosamine-induced liver injury in rats. *Bioscience, Biotechnology, and Biochemistry* 74, no. 3, 573–78.

Ayala, F., Kawanishi, K., Kuroiwa, E., Moriyasu, M., Tachibana, Y., Ueda, H. (2004). Aldose reductase inhibitors from the leaves of *Myrciaria dubia* (H. B. & K.) McVaugh. *Phytomedicine* 11, nos. 7–8, 652–56.

Bobbio, F. O., Cuevas, E., Mercadante, A. Z., Winterhalter, P., Zanatta, C. F. (2005). Determination of anthocyanins from camu-camu (*Myrciaria dubia*) by HPLC-PDA, HPLC-MS, and NMR. *Journal of Agricultural and Food Chemistry* 53, no. 24, 9531–35.

Bradfield, R. B., Roca, A. (1964). Camu-camu—a fruit high in ascorbic acid. *Journal of the American Dietetic Association* 44:28–30.

Da Silva, F., et al. (2005). Antigenotoxic effect of acute, subacute and chronic treatments with Amazonian camu-camu (*Myrciaria dubia*) juice on mice blood cells. *Food Chemistry and Toxicology* 50, no. 7, 2275–81.

Dib Taxi, C. M., de Menezes, H. C., Grosso, C. R., Santos, A. B. (2003). Study of the microencapsulation of camu-camu (*Myrciaria dubia*) juice. *Journal of Microencapsulation* 20, no. 4, 443–48.

Dufour, J. & Zapata, S. (1992). Camu-camu *Myrciaria dubia* (HBK) Mcvaugh: Chemical composition of fruit. *Journal of the Science of Food and Agriculture* 61, no. 3.

Evelázio de Souza, N., Justi, K. C., Matsushita, M., Visentainer, J. V. (2000). Nutritional composition and vitamin C stability in stored camu-camu (*Myrciaria dubia*) pulp. *Archivos Latinoamericanos de Nutrición* 50, no. 4, 405–8.

Franco, M. R. & Shibamoto, T. (2000). Volatile composition of some Brazilian fruits: umbu-caja (Spondias citherea), camu-camu (*Myrciaria dubia*), Araça-boi (*Eugenia stipitata*), and Cupuaçu (*Theobroma grandiflorum*). *Journal of Agricultural and Food Chemistry* 48, no. 4, 1263–65.

Genovese, M., Goncalves, A., Lajolo, F. (2010). Chemical composition and antioxidant/antidiabetic potential of Brazilian native fruits and commercial frozen pulps. *Journal of Agricultural & Food Chemistry* 58, no. 8.

Inoue, T., Komoda, H., Node, K., Uchida, T. (2008). Tropical fruit camu-camu (*Myrciaria dubia*) has anti-oxidative and anti-inflammatory properties. *Journal of Cardiology* 52, no. 2, 127–32.

Komoda, H., Inoue, T., Node, K., Uchida, T. (2008). Tropical fruit camu-camu (*Myrciaria dubia*) has anti-oxidative and anti-inflammatory properties. *Journal of Cardiology* 52.

Mazza, G. (2007). Anthocyanins and heart health. *Ann Ist Super Sanità* 43, no. 4, 369–74. Available at http://www.eatris.it/binary/publ/cont/369%20-20ANN_07_54_Mazza.1201593082.pdf.

Muller, V. (2010). Camu-camu (*Myrciaria dubia*). Whole World Botanicals. Retrieved from http://wholeworldbotanicals.com/herbal_camucamu.

Tohi, W. (2012). The true history of camu camu, nature's most potent source of natural vitamin C. Retrieved from http://www.naturalnews.com/037389_camu_history_vitamin_C.html.

Yazawa, K., et al. (2011). Anti-inflammatory effects of seeds of the tropical fruit camu-camu (*Myrciaria dubia*). *Journal of Nutritional Science and Vitaminology (Tokyo)* 57, no. 1, 104–7.

Chia Seeds

Ali, N. M., Beh, B. K., Ho, W. Y., Tan, S. G., Tan, S. K., Yeap, S. K. (2012). The promising future of Chia, *Salvia hispanica* L. *Journal of Biomedicine and Biotechnology* 2012:1–9.

Barcelo-Coblijn, G., Murphy, E. J. (2009). Alpha-linolenic acid and its conversion to longer chain n-3 fatty acids: Benefits for human health and a role in maintaining tissue n-3 fatty acid levels. *Progress in Lipid Research* 48:355–74.

Guevara-Cruz, M., Tovar, A., Aguilar-Salinas, C., Medina-Vera, I., Gil-Zenteno, L., Hernandez-Viveros, I., Lopez-Romero, P., Ordaz-Nava, G., Canizales-Quinteros, S., Guillen Pineda, L., Torres, N. (2012). A dietary pattern including nopal, chia seed, soy protein, and oat reduces serum triglycerides and glucose intolerance in patients with metabolic syndrome. *Journal of Nutrition* 142, no. 1, 64–69.

Patel, V., Preedy, V., Watson, R. (2011). "Whole and Ground Chia (*Salvia hispanica* L.) Seeds, Chia Oil: Effects on Plasma Lipids and Fatty Acids." In *Nuts and Seeds in Health and Disease Prevention*, chapter 37, 309–15.

Cilantro

Aissaoui, A., Israili, Z. H., Lyoussi, B., Zizi, S. (2011). Hypoglycemic and hypolipidemic effects of *Coriandrum sativum* L. in Meriones shawi rats. *Journal of Ethnopharmacology* 137, no. 1, 652–61.

Anton, L., Codiță, I., Coldea, I. L., Dobre, E., Drăgulescu, E. C., Drăcea, N. O., Dra-gomirescu, C. C., Lixandru, B. E., Rovinaru, C. (2010). Antimicrobial activity of plant essential oils against bacterial and fungal species involved in food poisoning and/or food decay. *Roumanian Archives of Microbiology and Immunology* 69, no. 4, 224–30.

Anuradha, C. V. & Deepa, B. (2011). Antioxidant potential of *Coriandrum sativum* L. seed extract. *Indian Journal of Experimental Biology* 49, no. 1, 30–38.

Devkar, R. V., Desai, S. N., Gandhi, H. P., Patel, D. K., Ramachandran, A. V. (2012). Cardio protective effect of *Coriandrum sativum* L. on isoproterenol-induced myocardial necrosis in rats. *Food and Chemical Toxicology* 50, no. 9, 3150–55.

Duarte, M. C., Duarte, R. M., Figueira, G. M., Furletti, V. F., Höfling, J. F., Mardegan. R. C., Obando-Pereda, G., Rehder, V. L., Sartoratto, A., Teixeira, I. P. (2011). Action of *Coriandrum sativum* L. essential oil upon oral candida albicans biofilm formation. *Evidenced Based Complementary Alternative Medicine*, May 21, 2011.

Ghorbani, A., Rakhshandeh, H., Sadeghnia, H. R. (2012). Sleep-prolonging effect of *Coriandrum sativum* hydro-alcoholic extract in mice. *Natural Product Research* 26, no. 22, 2095–98.

Inbavalli, R. & Sreelatha, S. (2012). Antioxidant, antihyperglycemic, and antihyperlipidemic effects of *Coriandrum sativum* leaf and stem in alloxan-induced diabetic rats. *Journal of Food Science* 77:119–23.

Kim, H. G., Kim, S. Y., Kim, Y. O., Oh, M. S., Park, G., Park, S. H. (2012). *Coriandrum sativum* L. protects human keratinocytes from oxidative stress by regulating oxidative defense systems. *Skin Pharmacology and Physiology* 25, no. 2, 93–99.

Cinnamon

Almér, L. O., Björgell, O., Darwiche, G., Hlebowicz, J. (2007). Effect of cinnamon on postprandial blood glucose, gastric emptying, and satiety in healthy subjects. *American Journal of Clinical Nutrition* 85, no. 6, 1552–56.

Food and Nutrition Board, Institute of Medicine. (2001). Dietary reference intakes for vitamin A, vitamin K, boron, chromium, copper, iodine, iron, manganese, molybdenum, nickel, silicon, vanadium, and zinc. Washington, DC: National Academy Press, 394–419.

Khan, A., Safdar, M., Ali Khan, M. M., Khattak, K. N., Anderson, R. A. (2003). Cinnamon improves glucose and lipids of people with type 2 diabetes. *Diabetes Care* 26, no. 12, 3215–18.

Reavley, N. (1999). *The New Encyclopedia of Vitamins, Minerals, Supplements, and Herbs.* New York: M. Evans and Company.

Cumin

Agah, S., Taleb, A. M., Moeini, R., Gorji, N., Nikbakht, H. (2013). Cumin extract for symptom control in patients with irritable bowel syndrome: A case series. *Middle East Journal of Digestive Disease* 5, no. 4, 217–22.

Hardin, K., Leklem, J. E., Leonard, S. K. (2001). Vitamin B-6 content of spices. *Journal of Food Composition and Analysis* 14:163–67.

National Nutrient Database for Standard Reference. (2005). Full report (All Nutrients): 02009, Spices, chili powder. Agricultural Research Service United States Department of Agriculture, Release 26.

Curry

Balasubramanian, K. (2006). Molecular orbital basis for yellow curry spice curcumin's prevention of Alzheimer's disease. *Journal of Agricultural and Food Chemistry* 54, no. 10, 3512–20.

Bérubé-Parent, S., Diepvens, K., Joosen, A. M., Tremblay, A., Westerterp-Plantenga, M. (2006). Metabolic effects of spices, teas, and caffeine. *Physiology & Behavior* 89, no. 1, 85–91.

Villegas, I., Sánchez-Fidalgo, S., Alarcón de la Lastra, C. (2008). New mechanisms and therapeutic potential of curcumin for colorectal cancer. *Molecular Nutrition & Food Research* 52, no. 9, 1040–61.

Kañiwa

Akesson, B., Alvarado, J. A., Bergenstahl, B., Penarrieta, J. M. (2008). Total antioxidant capacity and content of flavo-noids and other phenolic compounds in canihua (*Chenopodium pallidicaule*): An Andean pseudocereal. *Molecular Nutrition & Food Research* 52, no. 6, 708–17.

"Calories in Kañiwa." (n.d.). Calorie Count. Retrieved from http://caloriecount.about.com/calories-roland-kaniwa -i266353.

Espinoza, C., Jacobsen, S. E., Repo-Carrasco, R. (2003). Nutritional value and use of the Andean crops quinoa (*Chenopo-dium quinoa*) and kañiwa (*Chenopodium pallidicaule*). *Food Reviews International* 19, nos. 1–2, 179–89.

Repo-Carrasco-Valencia, R., Acevedo de La Cruz, A., Icochea Alvarez, J. C., Kallio, H. (2009). Chemical and functional characterizations of Kañiwa (*Chenopodium pallidicaule*) grain, extrudate and bran. *Plant Foods for Human Nutrition* 64, no. 2, 94–101.

Repo-Carrasco-Valencia, R., Encina, C. R., Binaghi, M. J., Greco, C. B., Ronayne de Ferrer, P. A. (2010). Effects of roasting and boiling of quinoa, kiwicha and kañiwa on composition and availability of minerals in vitro. *Journal of Food Agriculture* 90:2068–73.

Kiwicha

Amaya-Farfán, J. & Caselato-Sousa, V. (2012). State of knowledge on amaranth grain: A comprehensive review. *Journal of Food Science* 77, no. 4.

Bavec, F., Bavec, M., Jakop, M., Mlakar, S., Turinek, M. (2010). Grain amaranth as an alternative perspective crop in temperate climate. *Journal of Geography* 5, no. 1, 135–45.

National Nutrient Database for Standard Reference. (2005). Full report (All Nutrients): 20002, Amaranth grain, cooked. Agricultural Research Service United States Department of Agriculture, Release 26.

Lucuma

Apostolidis, E., Genovese, M. I., Lajolo, F. M., Pinto, Mda S., Ranilla, L. G., Shetty, K. (2009). Evaluation of antihyper-glycemia and antihypertension potential of native Peruvian fruits using in vitro models. *Journal of Medicinal Food* 12:278–91.

Chen, S. S., Datta, N., Jiang, Y. M., Shi, J., Tomás-Barberán, F. A., Singanusong, R., Yao, L. H. (2004). Flavonoids in food and their health benefits. *Plant Foods for Human Nutrition* 5:113–22.

Dini, I. (2011). Flavonoid glycosides from *Pourteria obovata* (R. Br.) fruit flour. *Food Chemistry* 124:884–88.

Rojo, L. E., Villano, C. M., Joseph, G., Schmidt, B., Shulaev, V., Shuman, J. L., Lila, M. A., Raskin, I. (2011). Wound-healing properties of nut oil from *Pouteria lucuma*. *Journal of Cosmetic Dermatology* 9, no. 3, 185–95.

Maca

Angeles, F., Condezo, L., Lao, J., Melchor, V., Miller, M., Okuhama, N., Sandoval, M. (2001). Antioxidant activity of cruciferous vegetable Maca (*Lepidium meyenii*). *Food Chemistry* 79, no. 2.

Bianchi, A. (2003). MACA *Lepidium meyenii*. *Boletín Latinoamericano y del Caribe de Plantas Medicinales y Aromáticas* 2, no. 3.

Cordova, A., Chung, A., Gonzales, C., Gonzales, G., Vega, K., Villena, A. (2001). *Lepidium meyenii* (maca) improved semen parameters in adult men. *Asian Journal of Andrology* 3.

Gonzales-Castaneda, C., Gonzales, C., Gonzales, G. F. (2009) *Lepidium meyenii* (maca): A plant from the highlands of Peru—from tradition to science [Abstract]. *Research in Complementary Medicine* 16, no. 6.

Gonzales, G. (2011). Ethnobiology and ethnopharmacology of *Lepidium meyenii* (maca), a plant from the Peruvian Highlands. *Evidence-Based Complementary and Alternative Medicine* 2012.

Kilham, C. (n.d.). "Maca: Peru's natural viagra." Retrieved from http://www.macaex.com/pdfs/Maca-Perus-Natural -Viagra-By-Chris-kilham_en.pdf.

Sandoval, M., et al. (2002). Antioxidant activity of the cruciferous vegetable Maca (*Lepdidium meyenii*). *Food Chemistry* 79:207–13.

Taylor, L. (2005). Maca (*Lepidium meyenii*). Retrieved from http://www.rain-tree.com/maca.htm.

Wang, Y., et al. (2007). Maca: An Andean crop with multi-pharmacological functions. *Food Research International* 40:783–92.

Papaya

Curb, D., Rodriguez, B., Willcox, B. (2008). Antioxidants in cardiovascular health and disease: Key lessons from epidemiologic studies. *American Journal of Cardiology* 101.

Hernandez, C. & Hernandez, M. (2012). "Papaya Power." Retrieved from http://www.pacificnaturopathic.com/articles/papaya_power.html.

Hewavitharana, A., Nguyen, T., Parat, M.-O., Shaw, P. (2013). Anticancer activity of *Carica papaya*: A review. *Molecular Nutrition & Food Research* 57:153–64.

Ortega, M. (2012). "Effect of proteolytic enzyme and fiber of papaya fruit on human digestive health." Retrieved from University of Illinois Dissertations and Theses.

Paprika

Hautvast, J. G., van Het Hof, K. H., West, C. E., Weststrate, J. A. (2003). Dietary factors that affect the bioavailability of carotenoids. *Journal of Nutrition* 130, no. 3, 503–6.

Institute of Medicine, Food and Nutrition Board. (2000). "Beta-Carotene and Other Carotenoids." In *Dietary Reference Intakes for Vitamin C, Vitamin E, Selenium, and Carotenoids*. Washington, DC: National Academy Press, 325–400.

Minguez-Mosquera, M. I. & Hornero-Mendez, D. (1994). Comparative study of the effect of paprika processing on the carotenoids in peppers (*Capsicum annuum*) of the Bola and Agridulce varieties. *Journal of Agricultural and Food Chemistry* 42:1555–60.

Pichuberry

Aggarwal, B., Ichikawa, H., Jayaprakasam, B., Nair, M., Shishodia, T., Takada, Y. (2006). Withanolides potentiate apoptosis, inhibit invasion, and abolish osteoclastogenesis through suppression of nuclear factor-KB (NF-KB) activation and NF-KB-regulated gene expression. *Molecular Cancer Therapeutics* 5, no. 6.

Arun, M. & Asha, V. V. (2007). Preliminary studies on antihepatotoxic effect of *Physalis peruviana* Linn (Solanaceae) against carbon tetrachloride induced acute liver injury in rats. *Journal of Ethnopharmacology* 111, no. 1, 110–14.

Fang, S. T., Liu, J. K., Li, B. (2012). Ten new withanolides from *Physalis peruviana*. *Steroids* 77:36–44.

Fischer, G., Ebert, G., Ludders, P. (2000). Provitamin A carotenoids, organic acids and ascorbic acid content of cape gooseberry (*Physalis peruviana* L.) ecotypes grown at two tropical altitudes. *Acta Horticulturae* 351:263–68.

Franco, L. A., Matiz, G. E., Calle, J., Pinzon, R., Ospina, L. F. (2007). Actividad antinflamatoria de extractos y fracciones obtenidas de calices de *Physalis peruviana* L. *Biomedica* 47, no. 1, 51–60.

Martínez, W., Ospina, L. F., Granados, D., Delago, G. (2010). In vitro studies on the relationship between the anti-inflammatory activity of *Physalis peruviana* extracts and the phagocytic process. *Immunopharmacology and Immunotoxicology* 32, no. 1, 63–73.

Puente, L. A., Pinto-Munoz, C. A., Castro, E. S., Cortes, M. (2011). *Physalis peruviana* Linnaeus, the multiple properties of a highly functional fruit: A review. *Food Research International* 44:1733–40.

Ramadan, M. F. & Morsel, J. T. (2003). Oil Goldenberry (*Physalis peruviana* L.). *Journal of Agriculture and Food Chemistry* 51, no. 4, 969–74.

———. (2005). Cape gooseberry: A golden fruit of golden future. *Fruit Processing* 15, no. 6, 396–400.

Rockenbach, I. I. et al. (2008). Phenolic acids and antioxidant activity of *Physalis peruviana* L. fruit. *Alimentos e Nutricao* 19, no. 3, 271–76.

Wu, S. J. et al. (2005). Antioxidant activities of *Physalis peruviana*. *Biological Pharmaceutical Bulletin* 28, no. 6, 963–66.

Yen, C. Y. et al. (2010). 4B-Hydroxywithanolide E from *Physalis peruviana* (golden berry) inhibits growth of human lung cancer cells through DNA damage, apoptosis and G2/M arrest. *BMC Cancer* 10, no. 46.

Purple Corn

Jones, K. (2005). The potential health benefits of purple corn. *Herbal Gram* 65:46–49.

Kang, S. W., Kang, Y. H., Kim, J. K., Kim, J. L., Lee, J. Y., Li, J., Lim, S. S. (2012). Purple corn anthocyanins dampened high-glucose-induced mesangial fibrosis and inflammation: Possible renoprotective role in diabetic nephropathy. *Journal of Nutritional Biochemistry* 23:320–31.

Long, N., Naiki-ito, A., Sakatani, K., Sato, S., Shirai, T., Suzuki, S., Takahashi, S. (2013). Purple corn color inhibition of prostate carcinogenesis by targeting cell growth pathways. *Cancer Science* 104:298–303.

Mazza, G. (2007). Anthocyanins and heart health. *Ann Ist Super Sanità* 43:369–74.

Purple Potatoes

Furuta, S., Kobayashi, M., Masuda, M., Nishiba, Y., Oki, T., Suda, I. (2003). Physiological functionality of purple-fleshed sweet potatoes containing anthocyanins and their utilization in foods. *Japan Agricultural Research Quarterly* 73:167–73.

Galli, R., Joseph, J., Shukitt-Hale, B., Youdim, K. (2002). Fruit polyphenolics and brain agin. *Annals of New York Academy of Sciences* 959:128–32.

Hamouz, K. & Lachman, J. (2005). Red and purple coloured potatoes as a significant antioxidant source in human nutrition—a review. *Plant, Soil, and Environment* 51:477–82.

Makkieh, K. (n.d.). "Purple Potatoes Nutrition Facts." Healthy Eating. Retrieved from http://healthyeating.sfgate.com/purple-potatoes-nutrition-2182.html.

Mazza, G. (2007). Anthocyanins and heart health. *Ann Ist Super Sanità* 43:369–74.

Stoner, G. & Wang, L. (2008). Anthocyanins and their role in cancer prevention. *Cancer Letters* 269:281–90.

Quinoa

Espinoza, C., Jacobsen, S. E., Repo-Carrasco, R. (2003). Nutritional value and use of the Andean crops quinoa (*Chenopodium quinoa*) and kañiwa (*Chenopodium pallidicaule*). *Food Reviews International* 19, nos. 1–2, 179–89.

James, A. & Lilian, E. (2009). Quinoa (*Chenopodium quinoa* willd.): Composition, chemistry, nutritional, and functional properties. *Advances in Food and Nutrition Research* 58:1–31.

Martínez, E., Miranda, M., Puente, L., Uribe, E., Vega-Galvez, A., Vergara, J. (2010). Nutrition facts and functional potential of quinoa (*Chenopodium quinoa* willd.), an ancient Andean grain: A review. *Journal of the Science of Food and Agriculture* 90, no. 15, 2541–47.

Sacha Inchi

Beccaria, M., Cacciola, F., Dacha, M., Dugo, L., Dugo, P., Fanali, C., Mondello, L. (2011). Chemical characterization of sacha inchi (*plukenetia volubilis l.*) oil. *Journal of Agriculture and Food Chemistry* 59.

Cabo, N., Chirinos, R., Gloria, P., Guillen, M. (2003). Characterization of sacha inchi (*Plukenetia volubilis l.*) oil by FTIR spectroscopy and ^{1}H NMR: Comparison with linseed oil. *Journal of American Oil Chemists' Society* 80, no. 8.

Curb, D., Rodriguez, B., Willcox, B. (2008). Antioxidants in cardiovascular health and disease: Key lessons from epidemiologic studies. *American Journal of Cardiology* 10.

Gomez-Pinilla, F. (2011). Collaborative effects of diet and exercise on cognitive enhancement. *Nutrition and Health* 20.

Gutierrez, L., Jimenez, A., Rosada, L. (2010). Chemical composition of sacha inchi (*Plukenetia volubilis l.*) seeds and characteristics of their lipid fraction. *Instituto de Ciencia y Tecnologia de Alimentos (ICTA)* 30.

Pinilla, F. (2008). Brain foods: The effects of nutrients on brain function. *Nature Reviews of Neuroscience* 9.

Sweet Potatoes

Block, G. (1991). Vitamin C and cancer prevention: The epidemiologic evidence. *American Journal of Clinical Nutrition* 5, no. 1, 2705–2825.

Mayne, S. (1996). Beta-carotene, carotenoids, and disease prevention in humans. *Journal of the Federation of American Societies for Experimental Biology* 10:690–710.

Yanuq, S. A. C. (2008). "Sweet Potato." Yanuq. Retrieved from http://www.yanuq.com/english/Articulos_Publicados/sweetypotatoe.htm.

Turmeric

Ahsan, H., Hadi, S. M., Khan, N. U., Parveen, N. (1999). Pro-oxidant, anti-oxidant and cleavage activities on DNA of curcumin and its derivatives demethoxycurcumin and bisdemethoxycurcumin. *Chemico-Biological Interaction* 121, no. 2, 161–75.

Al-Delaimy, W. K., Heath, D. D., Rock, C. L., Tayyem, R. F. (2006). Curcumin content of turmeric and curry powders. *Nutrition & Cancer* 55, no. 2, 126–31.

Brouet, I. & Ohshima, H. (1995). Curcumin, an anti-tumour promoter and anti-inflammatory agent, inhibits induction of nitric oxide synthase in activated macrophages. *Biochemical & Biophysical Research Community* 206, no. 2, 533–40.

Butterfield, D. A., Calabrese, V., Stella, A. M. (2003). Nutritional antioxidants and the heme-oxygenase pathway of stress tolerance: Novel targets for neuroprotection in Alzheimer's disease. *Italian Journal of Biochemistry* 52, no. 4, 177–81.

Dai, Y., Dong, L., Jiang, X., Liang, G., Shan, X., Wu, J., Xu, F., Yang, S., Zhang, Y., Zhao, L., Zou, P. (2014). Synthesis and evaluation of a series of novel asymmetrical curcumin analogs for the treatment of inflammation. *Molecules* 19, no. 6, 7287–307.

Jurenka, J. S. (2009). Anti-inflammatory properties of curcumin, a major constituent of *Curcuma longa*: A review of preclinical and clinical research. *Alternative Medicine Review* 14, no. 2, 141–51.

Yacon

Andrade, A., Guerra, N., Livera, A., Padilha, V., Rolim, P., Salgado, S. (2011). Glycemic profile and prebiotic potential "in vitro" of bread with yacon (*Smallanthus sonchifolius*) flour. *Ciencia Y Tecnologia Alimentaria* 31, no. 2.

Fernández, M., Lachman, E. C., Orsák, M. (2003). Yacon [*Smallabthus sonchifolius* (Poepp. Et Endl.) H. Robinson] chemical composition and use: A review. *Plant, Soil, and Environment* 49:283–90.

Gorbach, S. (2000). Probiotics and gastrointestinal health. *American Journal of Gastroenterology* 95, no. 1, S2–S4.

Valentová, K. & Ulrichová, J. (2003). *Smallanthus sonchifolius* and *lepidium meyenii*—prospective Andean crops for the prevention of chronic diseases. *Biomedical Papers* 147, no. 2, 119–30.

Yuca

Bae, C. Y., Bae, D. H., Kang, H. C., Kang, S. I., Kim, S. W., Oh, H. J., Park, S. K. (2003). Hypocholesterolemic property of *Yucca schidigera* and *Quillaja saponaria* extracts in human body. *Archives of Pharmaceutical Research* 26:1042–46.

Cheeke, P. R., Oleszek, W., Piacente, S. (2006). Anti-inflammatory and anti-arthritic effects of *Yucca schidigera*: A review. *Journal of Inflammation* 3, no. 6, 1–7.

Olas, B., Oleszek, W., Stochmal, A., Wachowicz, B. (2003). Inhibition of oxidative stress in blood platelets by different phenolics from *Yucca schidigera* Roezl bark. *Nutrition* 19, no. 7, 633–40.

Other

"A Gastronomic Discovery of Peru | Discover South America." (n.d.). Epicurious Travel. Retrieved from http://www.epicurioustravel.com.au/journey/a-gastronomic-discovery-of-peru.

Alvarez-Dongo, D., Sanchez-Abanto, J., Gomez-Guizado, G., Tarqui-Mamani, C. (2009–2010) Overweight and Obesity: Prevalence and Determining Social Factors of Overwight in the Peruvian Population. *Revista Peruana de Medicina Experimental y Salud Publica*. 29, no. 3, 303-13.

Alzamora, S., Barbosa-Cánovas, G., Chanes, J., Fernández-Molina, J., López-Malo, A., Tapia, M. (2003). *Handling and Preservation of Fruits and Vegetables by Combined Methods for Rural Areas*. Food and Agriculture Organization of the United Nations: Technical Manual, Bulletin 49, Chapter 1.

American Diabetes Association. (2013). "Fast Facts: Data and Statistics about Diabetes." Retrieved from http://professional.diabetes.org/admin/UserFiles/0%20-%20Sean/FastFacts%20March%202013.pdf.

Arbanil-Huaman, H., Pajuelo-Ramirez, J., Sanchez-Abanto, J. (2010). Nontransmissible diseases in Peru and their relationship with altitude. *Revista de la Sociedad Peruana de Medicina Interna.* 23, no. 2, 45–51.

Bethene Ervin, R. (2009). Prevalence of metabolic syndrome among adults 20 years of age and over, by sex, age, race and ethnicity, and body mass index: United States, 2003–2006. National Health Statistics Report, US Department of Health and Human Resources, CDC, no. 13, 1–8.

Cardenas-Quintana, H., Mendozaq-Tasayco, F., Roldan-Arbieto, L., Sanchez-Abanto, J. (2009). Prevalence of Metabolic Syndrome in People 20 Years Old and More. *Revista Espanola de Salud Publica.* 83, no. 2, 257-265.

Centers for Disease Control and Prevention. (2014)."Obesity and Overweight." Retrieved from http://www.cdc.gov/nchs/fastats/obesity-overweight.htm.

Chase, R. (2013). "*USA Today* says Peruvian cuisine will be one of 2014's big food trends." Peru this Week website. Retrieved http://www.peruthisweek.com/news-usa-today-says-peruvian-cuisine-will-be-one-of-2014s-big-food-trends-101829.

Diabetes Prevalence—Country Rankings. (2010). Countries of the World website. Retrieved from http://www.allcountries.org/ranks/diabetes_prevalence_country_ranks.html.

Pajuelo-Ramirez, J., Sanchez-Abanto J. (2010). Adult nutritional status related to cardiovascular risk. *Revista de la Sociedad Peruana de Medicina Interna* 23, no. 3, 85–90.

Ramirez, J. & Sanchez, J. (2007). Adult metabolic syndrome in Peru. *Anales de la Facultad de Medicina* 68, no. 1, 38–46.

"2013 International Year of Quinoa." (2013). Quinoa 2013 International Year. Retrieved from http://www.rlc.fao.org/en/about-fao/iyq-2012/.

US Department of Health and Human Services. (n.d.). "About Overweight and Obesity Statistics." (n.d.). Retrieved from http://win.niddk.nih.gov/publications/PDFs/stat904z.pdf.

Walters, S. (2008). "The Healing Properties of Purple Corn." Natural News website. Retrieved from http://www.naturalnews.com/023800_purple_corn_blood_healing.html.

ABOUT THE AUTHOR

A nationally recognized, award-winning registered dietitian with more than sixteen years of experience as a nutritionist, **Manuel Villacorta, M.S., R.D.**, is a respected and trusted voice in the health and wellness industry. He is the founder of Eating Free, an international weight management and wellness program, and one of the leading weight loss and nutrition experts in the country. He is the author of *Eating Free: The Carb-Friendly Way to Lose Inches, Embrace Your Hunger, and Keep the Weight Off for Good* (HCI, May 2012) and *Peruvian Power Foods: 18 Superfoods, 101 Recipes, and Anti-Aging Secrets from the Amazon to the Andes* (HCI, October 2013). Manuel served as a national media spokesperson for the Academy of Nutrition and Dietetics (2010–13) and currently acts as a health blog contributor for the *Huffington Post*, an on-air contributor to the Univision television network, and a health and lifestyle contributor for *Fox News Latino* and *Peru This Week*. Manuel is a national spokesperson for the Pichuberry Company and for youthH20. Manuel is the owner of the San Francisco–based private practice MV Nutrition and is the recipient of five Best Bay Area Nutritionist awards (2008, 2009, 2010, 2012, and 2013) from the *San Francisco Chronicle*, *ABC7*, and *Citysearch*. His warm, approachable style and his bilingual proficiency in English and Spanish have made him an in-demand health and nutrition expert on local and national television and radio channels, as well as in articles appearing in print publications and online.

Born and raised in Peru, Manuel makes his home in San Francisco. He earned his bachelor of science in nutrition and physiology metabolism from the University of California, Berkeley, and his master of science in nutrition and food science from San Jose State University. He has been the recipient of numerous prestigious awards for his research and contributions to the field of dietetics.

ABOUT THE CONTRIBUTOR

Sarah Koszyk, M.A., R.D., is a national award–winning registered dietitian and nutrition therapist. Sarah works at the San Francisco–based private practice MV Nutrition, which follows the Eating Free national plan. She is a writer/contributor for various online outlets. She has brought warmth, compassion, and expertise to her clients in order for them to reach their nutrition, health, and weight goals. Sarah empowers her clients to know exactly what to do to maintain optimal health in a realistic, long-term, sustainable lifestyle approach.

With a passion for food and travel, Sarah has visited more than twenty-five countries around the world and spends at least two months traveling every year. Experiencing international cuisines and taking cooking classes in the various countries is one of her many enthusiasms. In addition, her love of scuba diving takes her on more adventures worldwide, where she thoroughly enjoys her time in the sea swimming with the fish.

INDEX